Healthcare Logistics and Supply Chain Management

From Foundation to Best Practices

Healthcare Logistics and Supply Chain Management

From Foundation to Best Practices

Duangpun Kritchanchai
Mahidol University, Thailand

Albert Wee Kwan Tan
Asia Institute of Management, Philippines

Sirirat Srisakunwan
Mahidol University, Thailand

World Scientific

NEW JERSEY • LONDON • SINGAPORE • BEIJING • SHANGHAI • HONG KONG • TAIPEI • CHENNAI • TOKYO

Published by

World Scientific Publishing Co. Pte. Ltd.

5 Toh Tuck Link, Singapore 596224

USA office: 27 Warren Street, Suite 401-402, Hackensack, NJ 07601

UK office: 57 Shelton Street, Covent Garden, London WC2H 9HE

Library of Congress Cataloging-in-Publication Data

Names: Kritchanchai, Duangpun author | Tan, Albert Wee Kwan, 1962– author | Srisakunwan, Sirirat author

Title: Healthcare logistics and supply chain management : from foundation to best practices / authors Duangpun Kritchanchai (Mahidol University, Thailand), Albert Wee Kwan Tan (Asia Institute of Management, Philippines), Sirirat Srisakunwan (Mahidol University, Thailand).

Description: New Jersey : World Scientific, [2027] | Includes bibliographical references and index.

Identifiers: LCCN 2026006260 | ISBN 9789819826155 hardcover | ISBN 9789819826162 ebook | ISBN 9789819826179 ebook other

Subjects: LCSH: Hospitals--Materials management | Hospital purchasing | Supply chain management

Classification: LCC RA971.33 .K75 2027

LC record available at https://lccn.loc.gov/2026006260

British Library Cataloguing-in-Publication Data

A catalogue record for this book is available from the British Library.

For any available supplementary material, please visit
https://www.worldscientific.com/worldscibooks/10.1142/14671#t=suppl

Desk Editors: Nambirajan Karuppiah/Pui Yee Lum

Typeset by Stallion Press
Email: enquiries@stallionpress.com

Preface

The healthcare industry is rapidly evolving, with logistics management playing a pivotal role in ensuring efficient and effective patient care. The intricacies of hospital logistics, ranging from inventory control to transportation management, require a comprehensive understanding and strategic approach. This book aims to elucidate these complexities and provide actionable insights into hospital logistics management.

Chapter 1: Foundations of Hospital Logistics Management

In this opening chapter, we delve into the fundamental components of hospital logistics systems. We explore the various nodes and links, materials management, and information management that form the backbone of a hospital's logistics network. This chapter also examines these systems, focusing on organization and staffing, warehousing and storage, inventory control processes, procurement, demand forecasting, logistics management information systems, and the transportation and distribution of products to service units or patients. By understanding these foundational elements, readers will gain a solid foundation in the essential aspects of hospital logistics management.

Chapter 2: Effective Inventory Management in Hospitals

Inventory management is a critical aspect of hospital logistics, ensuring that the right supplies are available when needed. This chapter presents an in-depth analysis of the types of inventories within the logistics system and addresses common inventory management challenges in hospitals. Through a detailed case study, we assess current ordering and inventory management processes, procedures, and tools used for calculations. We also introduce the design and development of a dashboard tailored for inventory management, backed by comprehensive data analysis. This chapter provides practical solutions and tools to improve inventory management efficiency in terms of both cost-effectiveness and accuracy.

Chapter 3: Optimizing Hospital Logistics Flows

Efficient management of logistics flows is vital for the smooth operation of hospital logistics. Chapter 3 focuses on the management of flow diagrams, facility layout, line balancing, and flow routing within a hospital setting. This chapter introduces innovative concepts, such as the establishment of a central warehouse serving multiples hospitals and the development of an in-warehouse platform system, aimed at enhancing hospital transportation management. These strategies are designed to streamline operations, reduce costs, and improve overall logistics efficiency.

Chapter 4: Action Plan for Enhancing Hospital Logistics

In this chapter, the chapter outlines a strategic action plan to enhance hospital logistics systems. We cover resource management, reverse logistics of drugs and medical supplies, and sub-action plans for material inventory management, transportation management, and the establishment of a logistics agency. The application of barcodes in hospital logistics systems is also discussed as a means to streamline processes and improve efficiency. By implementing these action plans, hospitals can achieve significant improvements in their logistics operations.

Chapter 5: Building Robust Logistics Infrastructure in Public Health Systems

This chapter examines the design and development of logistics infrastructure and integrated information systems. The chapter provides guidelines for healthcare big data as part of Thailand's Digital Economy initiative and present project case studies, including the development of a COVID-19 vaccine cold chain to ensure temperature control and traceability in transportation and storage. These case studies emphasize the importance of robust logistics infrastructure in maintaining the quality and safety of healthcare services.

Chapter 6: Cutting-Edge Research in Hospital Logistics

In Chapter 6, the chapter explore the application of new information technologies in hospital logistics. It discusses the creation of a simulation model for the allocation of service units in the outpatient department and present a case study on designing a porter management system within a hospital. This chapter showcases the latest research and technological advancements in hospital logistics, and provides insights into how these innovations can be applied to improve logistics management.

Chapter 7: Best Practices in Hospital Logistics Systems

The final chapter presents the results of studies on prototype logistics systems implemented across in 17 hospitals. The chapter highlight the lessons learned and identify key success factors, providing valuable insights for the development and improvement of logistics systems in healthcare facilities. By examining best practices and successful case studies, readers can gain practical knowledge and strategies for implementation in their respective hospital logistics operations.

This book is a culmination of extensive research, practical insights, and innovative solutions aimed at transforming hospital logistics management. It is intended to serve as a valuable resource for healthcare professionals, logisticians, and anyone involved in the complex yet essential field of hospital logistics.

About the Authors

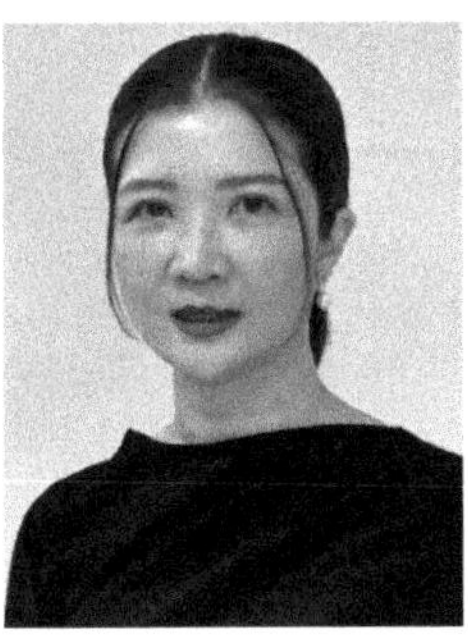

Duangpun Kritchanchai is an Associate Professor in the Department of Industrial Engineering at Mahidol University, where she also serves as the Director of the Centre of Logistics Management and Healthcare Supply Chain (LogHealth). She earned her PhD and master's degree in Manufacturing Engineering and Operations Management from the University of Nottingham, United Kingdom.

Her research portfolio is distinguished by a macroscopic focus on transforming national and regional healthcare systems through logistics and supply chain innovation. Dr Kritchanchai's work emphasizes the systemic improvement of healthcare operations, ranging from the development of national innovation networks to the design of integrated logistics frameworks for the public health sector. She has played a pivotal role in shaping healthcare supply chain policies and fostering connectivity within the ASEAN region to enhance overall system efficiency. Beyond academic excellence, her contributions focus on the strategic application of digital technology and standardization to improve service delivery on a large scale. As a prolific researcher, she has led numerous high-impact strategic projects and authored foundational textbooks that serve as key resources for the field of healthcare operations management.

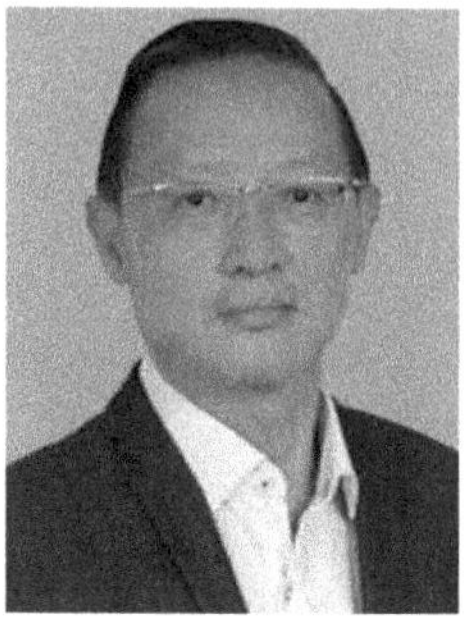

Albert Wee Kwan Tan joined the AIM faculty as an Associate Professor and Academic Program Director of the Online MBA program. He has a combined 32 years of industry practice and teaching experience in Australia, Singapore, China, Dubai, Indonesia, Malaysia, and Vietnam. Most recently, he was a visiting professor at NUS in Singapore, MIT SCALE Network, Wollongong in Dubai, Curtin in Australia, as well as in Indonesia and Vietnam.

Dr Tan was conferred a bachelor's in Information Technology in 1996 by the University of Southern Queensland. He also obtained a master's in Business Studies from the University of Ireland in 1998 and a PhD in Operations Management from Nanyang Technological University in 2005. He is also a certified Fellow in Production and Inventory Management (CPIM-F) from APICS.

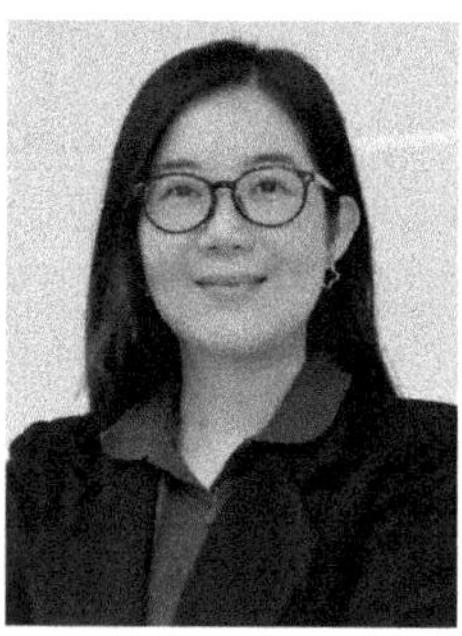

Sirirat Srisakunwan is a researcher at the Centre of Logistics Management and Healthcare Supply Chain (LogHealth), Faculty of Engineering, Mahidol University. She holds a Master of Management (Dean's List with Distinction) and a Bachelor of Engineering in Industrial Engineering from Mahidol University. With over 15 years of combined experience in both academia and the automotive and electronic industries, she possesses a unique ability to bridge theoretical frameworks with practical, large-scale industrial applications.

Her research portfolio focuses on the systemic transformation of healthcare infrastructure through logistics innovation and digital integration. Sirirat has been a key contributor to significant national-level projects, including the design of logistics frameworks for geriatric medicine, the development of vaccine cold chain management systems during the pandemic, and the strategic implementation of Big Data initiatives for Thailand's digital health economy. Her work emphasizes enhancing public health resilience by integrating emerging technologies such as RFID and AI into supply chain operations. As an author and consultant, she has published extensively on supply chain resilience and frequently shares her expertise as a lecturer for national healthcare accreditation bodies.

Contents

Glossary of Key Terms

The terms below are defined in accordance with established literature and widely accepted industry standards.

ABC Analysis—A method of classifying inventory into three categories (A, B, C) based on importance, usage, or value, often using the Pareto principle (80/20 rule) (Silver, Pyke, & Thomas, 2016).

Bullwhip Effect—A supply chain phenomenon where small fluctuations in demand at the consumer level cause larger variations upstream in procurement, production, and distribution (Lee, Padmanabhan, & Whang, 1997).

Cold Chain—A temperature-controlled supply chain system for storing, transporting, and distributing temperature-sensitive products such as vaccines, blood, and medicines (Chen *et al.*, 2023).

Distribution Center (DC)—A facility where products are received, stored, and redistributed to hospitals, clinics, or pharmacies (Chopra & Meindl, 2016).

Economic Order Quantity (EOQ)—A formula that determines the optimal order quantity to minimize total inventory costs, balancing holding costs and ordering costs (Harris, 1913).

First-Expired, First-Out (FEFO)—An inventory management method ensuring that items with the earliest expiry dates are used first (Dobson, Pinker, & Yurtseven, 2017).

Hospital Logistics—The management of the flow of medicines, equipment, consumables, and information within a hospital to ensure timely and efficient patient care (Volland *et al.*, 2017).

Inventory Turnover—A measure of how many times inventory is sold or used in a given period. High turnover often indicates efficient management (Muller, 2011).

Logistics Management Information System (LMIS)—A digital system for recording, tracking, and managing stock levels, distribution, and procurement in healthcare facilities (Kritchanchai, Hoeur, & Engelseth, 2018).

Order-up-to Level Policy—An inventory replenishment method where stock is ordered to reach a pre-set maximum level whenever it drops below a threshold (Axsäter, 2006).

Outpatient Department (OPD)—A hospital department where patients receive medical care without being admitted overnight (Cayirli & Veral, 2003).

Pareto Principle (80/20 Rule)—A concept where 20% of inputs or items account for 80% of results or value, commonly applied in inventory management (ABC classification) (Sanders, 1987).

Porter System—A logistics system in hospitals where designated staff (porters) transport patients, specimens, equipment, and supplies between departments (Odegaard *et al.*, 2007).

Supply Chain Resilience—The capacity of a healthcare supply chain to adapt, respond, and recover quickly from disruptions such as pandemics or natural disasters (Ivanov, 2020).

Chapter 1

Foundations of Hospital Logistics Management

A supply chain describes the interconnected movement of materials, products, and information that flows through various key players, which include manufacturers, sellers, distributors, customers, and consumers. These key players are linked through different business activities, such as procurement or purchasing, production or manufacturing, storage, IT, distribution, and transportation (Jüttner *et al.*, 2010).

Logistics is concerned with the strategic planning, execution, and management of the movement and storage of goods and services. It encompasses all aspects, from inbound and outbound transportation to the warehousing of products and information handling. The objective is to ensure seamless and effective operations from inception to completion. The objective is to meet customer requirements regarding delivery timing and more, production quality and quantity, cost efficiency, and delivery location (Bowersox, 2012). Figure 1.1 shows a supply chain with the information flow and material flow.

A Patient safety, an essential aspect of medical practice, focuses on the prevention of errors throughout each stage of the treatment process.

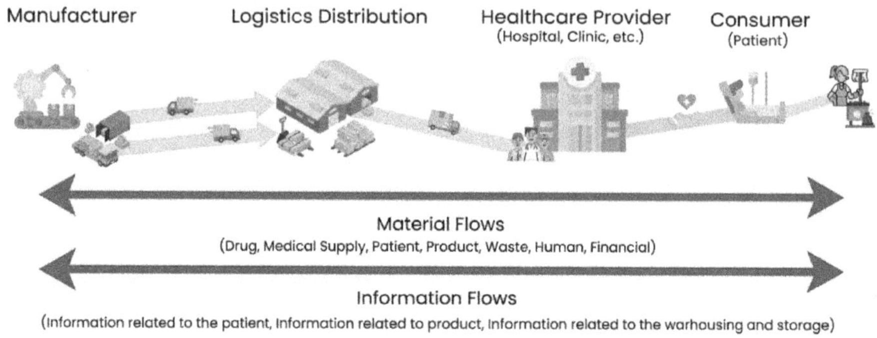

Figure 1.1. Supply chain, illustrating the journey of materials, products, information, and transactions from their starting point to their required destination.

A hospital is an institution providing essential medical materials, including medicines, supplies, and equipment, which significantly affects patients' lives. However, the complex flow of materials, people, and information within hospitals can lead to communication inefficiencies between departments. This complexity can make it difficult to effectively track and trace drugs and medical supplies during product issues or recalls.

Logistics is a process that involves three main flows. As defined by Stock and Lambert (2001), these flows take three primary forms:

1. Material flow (e.g., products and services) represents the physical movement of goods.
2. Information flow refers to the exchange of essential details neccesary for coordination, including the required product, its quantity, cost, and so forth.
3. Financial flow involve the transfer of funds or other forms of payment for goods or services. The main focus of this flow is on the product or service, with the objective of ensuring financial effective and transactional. Figure 1.2 illustrates the setup of a logistics system that encompasses 13 activities to facilitate this.

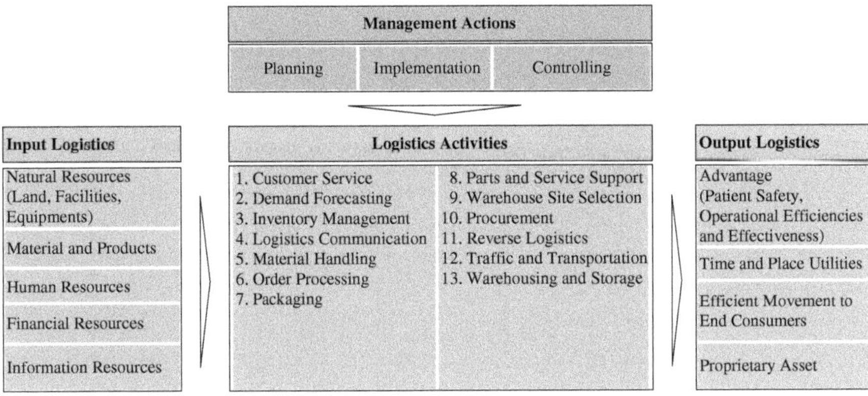

Figure 1.2. The 13 fundamental activities of a logistics system.

1.1 Components of Hospital Logistics Systems

This section explores hospital logistics systems, concentrating on two main areas: operations management and information management.

In evaluating the health logistics systems across hospitals of various sizes, from large medical centers to midsize community hospitals and smaller subdistrict health promotion hospitals, three main elements can be identified. These are (1) flow management (such as nodes & links), (2) resource management, and (3) information management.

1.1.1. Nodes and links: In the discussion of logistics, logistics systems can be simplified by identifying two key elements: nodes and links.

In the hospital context, a node represents any location, as shown in Figure 1.3, serving as a staging point, storage point,or distribution point. Examples include a drug warehouse, medical supply warehouse, ward, central distribution unit, laundry department, or nutrition department, among others.

In node management, the objective is to manage resource effectively across all functional areas. This encompasses warehouse management, where we optimize storage space is optimized; inventory management, where optimal stock levels are maintained; and capacity management, where appropriate capacity levels are determined.

A link refers to operations involving movement from one node to another, including a wide range of products. These movements may include the transportation of medicines, medical supplies, specimens, linen, food, and even waste materials, among other things.

Link management plays a key role in guiding the flow of transportation activities. This involves tasks such as establishing transportation paths (Routing), devising transport timetables (Scheduling), and organizing queues (Queuing), among other operational activities.

Information flow serves as a bridge between nodes and links within the hospital information systems. Generally, hospitals utilize two primary information systems: the front-end system and the back-end system. The front-end system is dedicated to patient services, including prescription processing, medication dispensing, and financial transactions. Conversely, the back-end system is primarily concerned with resource management, handling areas such as drug and medical supply inventory management. Connectivity is a critical aspect of information system governance. Specifically, the front-end

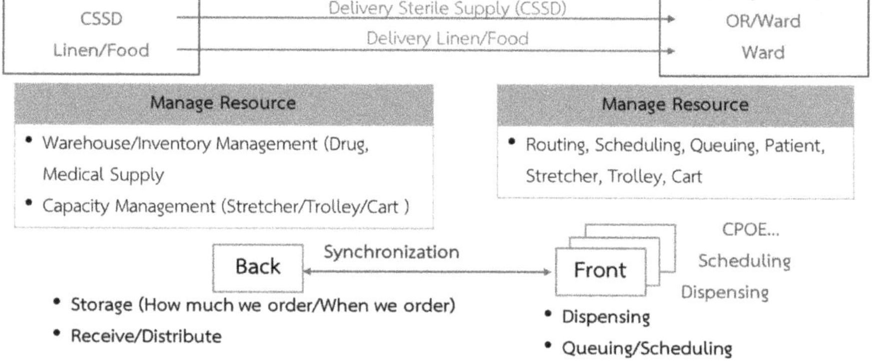

Figure 1.3. Features of nodes and links in hospitals logistics system (Kritchanchai & Srisakunwan, 2023a).

system should be synchronized with the back-end system to establish a unified data flow and manage data integration for effective collaboration.

1.1.2. Materials management: Materials, or goods, refer to items or entities that move within the logistics process to deliver services or support tasks. Through the effective management of these flows, hospital are able to fulfill their core mission. These items can be categorized into three main groups: patients, products, and waste, 8 as detailed further.

Patient The term "patient" refers to a wide variety of individuals. This includes outpatients receiving services, inpatients, maternity patients, and those transferred from network hospitals. It also encompasses patients referred to other healthcare facilities for specialized treatment.

Product "Product" refers to medicines, patient food, non-drug medical supplies, dental materials, autopsy materials, general medical supplies, medical equipment, sterile medical supplies, linen, and various office supplies.

Waste There are various types of waste, including general waste, infectious waste, and recyclable waste.

1.1.3. Information management: In the hospital logistics process, information is interconnected and influences product movement. Information is crucial for managing hospital operations. Generally, hospital logistics information can be classified into two categories details related to patients and information regarding products, as outlined below:

Information related to a patient This refers to data directly associated with the patient, such as details in the patient's medical records. Examples include laboratory test results, X-ray findings, and specifics of prescribed medications, among other clinical information.

Information related to a product This includes details related to the product, such as inventory balance and quality status. It also encompasses goods picking information, requisitions for medicines and medical supplies, and transfers document (e.g., waybill) between various service units.

1.2 Analysis of Hospital Logistics Systems

Supply chain management principles focus on strategically planning and managing activities and resources throughout the system. As such, they provide a useful lens for examining the management of hospital logistics systems in Thailand from a system analysis perspective. Hospital logistics can be segmented into seven distinct areas, each offering two analytical dimensions:

(1) Organization and Staffing,
(2) Warehousing and Storage,
(3) Inventory Control Processes,
(4) Procurement and Supply Chain Management,
(5) Forecasting,
(6) Logistics Management Information System, and
(7) Transportation and Distribution.

We can summarize a two-dimensional analysis of seven aspects of hospital logistics systems as depicted in Figure 1.4.

1.2.1. Organization and staffing: Personnel play a vital role in managing the logistics process. Under this study framework, logistics tasks encompass activities such as product selection, vendor evaluation, and price negotiation, as well as planning for product use and procurement and demand forecasting product usage. The process also includes product storage and distribution to end users. It is essential to maintain tools and equipment, such as product shelves, carts, and thermometers, ensuring their operational readiness at all time.

In many hospitals, logistics tasks are not consolidated under a single department. Instead, relevant operations such as product selection, procurement, maintenance, and distribution fall under the responsibility of the respective departments oversea those items. For instance, the pharmaceutical department handles logistics for drugs and non-drug medical supplies. Similarly, dental materials are

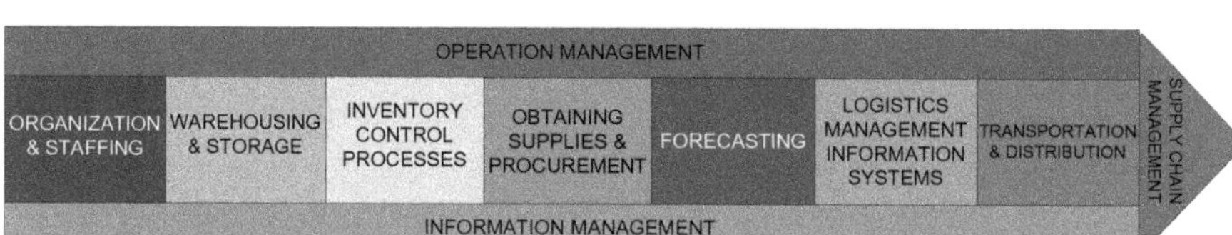

Figure 1.4. Seven aspects of hospital logistics management.

managed by the dental unit, materials used in the medical technology laboratory are overseen by the autopsy room, and the general administration department takes charge of equipment and office supplies.

The transportation division plans and controls the distribution of hospital supplies and materials. This includes the service support team, which effectively oversees the movement and transportation tailored to the type of product. For example, ward staff manage the collection of medicines and medical supplies according to physician's prescriptions, as well as other general medical supplies. Meanwhile, the laundry unit gathers used garments and ensures their proper laundering.

According to the organizational structure, most hospitals feature a management committee led by the director, with heads of various work groups serving as committee members. This committee is charged with the essential task of considering budget allocations for various purchases, including but not limited to medical supplies, non-medical materials, dental materials, autopsy materials, office supplies, and other equipment. Regularly scheduled meetings are held at regular intervals, allowing for the adjustment of purchase plans to reflect current circumstances.

1.2.2. Warehousing and storage: This refers to the task of managing storage space to preserve inventory and ensure its readiness for use.This entails managing product storage, warehouse space, and the upkeep of equipment and tools. It also includes various activities within the warehouse, such as receiving goods, inspecting products, maintaining inventory balance, and handling the disbursement and return of goods.

The majority of hospitals have dedicated storage spaces or warehouses for various items. These spaces are typically secure and monitored for the proper storage of goods. Detailed records of product receipts, payments, and current inventory levels are maintained at all times.

The warehouses can generally be classified into two categories:

(1) Medical supply warehouses: These store drugs, non-drug medical supplies, dental materials, and autopsy materials.
(2) General supply warehouses: These are meant for storing office supplies, housekeeping items, and kitchen goods.

Hospital warehouse can further be categorized as standalone warehouses or decentralized (Separate) warehouses, as illustrated in Figure 1.5.

Stand-alone warehouse	This is a warehouse that directly distributes products to end-users. It does not have any subsidiary depots or temporary storage points such as medical supply warehouses for drugs, medical supplies, and materials. It typically includes storage areas for reserve stock, office supply and housekeeping.
Separate warehouse	This is a warehouse that carries out identical functions to a stand-alone warehouse, yet it incorporates additional subdepots or stop points before the products reach the end-user. Examples of distinct warehouses within a hospital setting include medical supply warehouses for pharmaceuticals and prescribed medical supplies. Besides the main warehouse, there are also reserves of medicines and medical supplies located in outpatient and inpatient medication rooms, forming part of the supply chain before the final delivery to the service recipients.

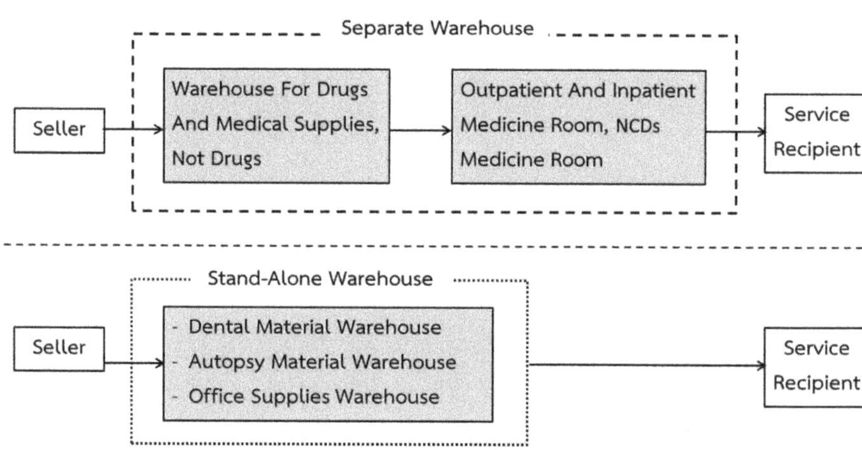

Figure 1.5. Overview of the physical attributes of hospital warehouses. (Kritchanchai & Srisakunwan, 2023a).

Table 1.1. Functions and responsibilities of hospital warehouses.

Warehouse	Functions and Responsibilities
Medical supply warehouse	• Manages the storage of various types of medicines, including liquids, tablets, injections, creams, and drugs, that require temperature control. Special attention should be given to narcotics, psychotropic drugs, and life-saving medications. • Maintains supplies of non-pharmaceutical medical items, including saline, cotton, gel, and wound cleanser. • Maintains an inventory of medical supplies, including items like test tubes, masks, syringes, and needle heads. • Maintains materials utilized in dental practices. • Manages materials used in medical technology laboratories, such as blood collection tubes and analytical reagents.
Parcel warehouse	Manages the office supplies and equipment, including cleaning solutions. Maintains records of the spare parts used for maintenance.

The roles and duties of the hospital warehouse are outlined in Table 1.1.

The primary responsibilities of the warehouse include inspecting incoming goods, conducting physical quality checks, storage, and distribution to end users. This also involves frequent inventory checks, such as weekly or monthly, to ensure the accurate balance of products. Every detail is precisely recorded during the receiving and disbursement processes. This includes the product name, requested quantity and unit for withdrawal, production lot number, and the product's expiration date.

It has been observed that our current product balance tracking system, i.e., on-hand inventory can only monitor products housed in the main warehouse. When items are allocated from the main warehouse, the system promptly subtracts from the remaining balance within the information system. This occurs even when the product has not been utilized yet. Consequently, the product balance displayed in the information system only reflects those items stored in the main warehouse. For further details, refer to Figure 1.6.

1.2.3. Inventory control processes: Inventory management is a vital activity, particularly in a hospital setting where the quantity

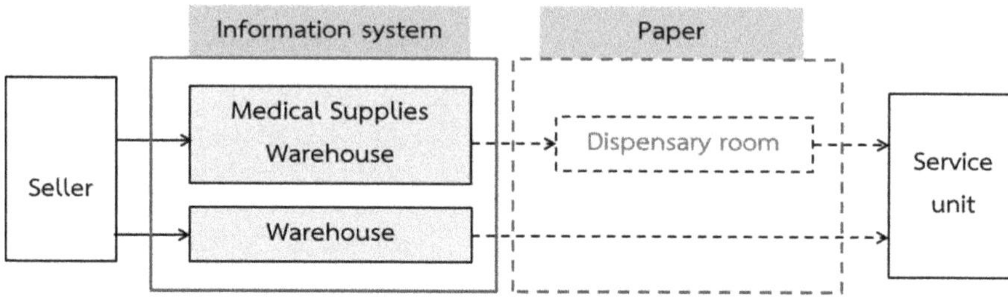

Figure 1.6. Division of information systems for managing inventory (Kritchanchai & Srisakunwan, 2023a).

of goods directly impacts the available funds. Maintaining an adequately stocked inventory is essential for meeting the needs of service recipients. However, a large reserve can also tie up capital, preventing its use in other areas of the hospital. Furthermore, these products' storage costs can add up. Therefore, keeping an appropriate balance in maintaining inventory levels to meet service needs with in a reasonable cost is essential in today's hospital management.

Typically, hospitals maintain reserve inventories in six categories:

1. Drugs,
2. Medical supplies, not drug,
3. Medical materials,
4. Dental materials,
5. Autopsy materials, and
6. Office supplies.

The product categories with no reserves include clothing and patient food ingredients. In addition, there is a minimal reserve for office supplies, as they are usually purchased locally on an as-needed basis. When products are received, they are promptly delivered to the designated service recipient.

Inventory coverage typically ranges from 1.5 to 2 months, depending on the product group within the hospital. This duration is necessary to adequately cater to the needs of service recipients, as well as to account for potential variations in the seller's product delivery.

However, we have observed instances of product shortages, returns, and exchanges with sellers. These situations often arise due to product deterioration or expired products. This is largely due to the decentralized nature of hospital inventory, which is spread across various locations such as the main warehouse, dispensary room, and patient wards. This distribution method is intended to meet demand in a timely manner.

Hospital inventory management is organized into two categories: prescription products and reserve products. The details are as follows:

Prescription products	Managing drugs, medical supplies, and office supplies forms a crucial part of our operation. This includes items such as alcohol, gloves, hand sanitizing gel, and office supplies. These are withdrawn by the service unit as per operational needs.
Reserve products	Goods are selected for patient use on a daily basis according to prescriptions. The frequency of restocking depends on an agreement between the warehouse and the service unit, establishing withdrawal days and times.

In terms of product distribution, a person in charge or a service team would make a request, specifying the quantity of goods needed for each order. This decision is influenced by historical usage patterns, current demand, inventory on hand, and other relevant factors. For instance, an anticipated increase in patients requiring specific pharmaceutical supplies may prompt them to maintain additional stock.

When distributing products, adhere to the product picking slip on an individual basis (Order Picking). Refrain from stacking all the product picking slips together for a single pickup. The process for product distribution is illustrated in Figure 1.7.

Inventory counting is the process of comparing the number of stock items recorded in the information system to the actual quantity present in the warehouse. In situations where the warehouse lacks an information system, the product control account can serve as a reliable tool for these comparisons, thus reducing the frequency of physical counts.

Notably, no clustering technique has been implemented so far. The ABC product movement does not contribute to product counting in

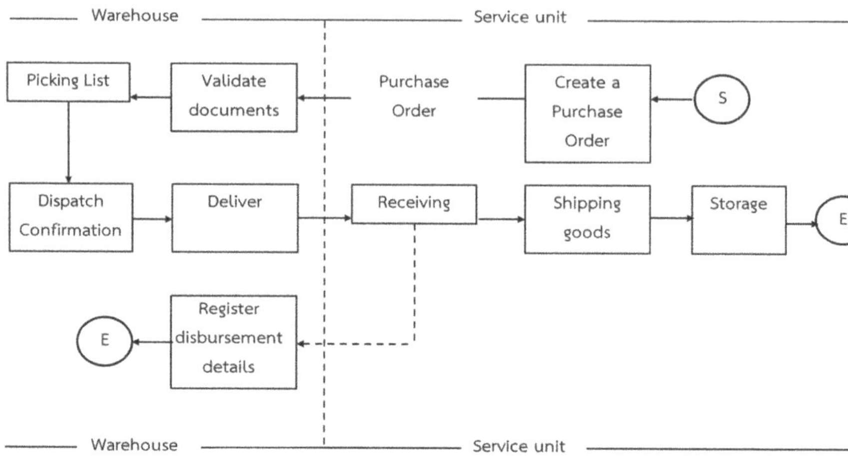

Figure 1.7. The hospital's product disbursement process.

any significant way. The hospital conducts annual product counts in accordance with the regulations of the Comptroller General's Department. When there is a discrepancy between the physical stock and the inventory in the computer system, an end-of-year report must be submitted to the committee. This committee investigates the cause and recommends improvements or other appropriate measures to enhance inventory balance.

1.2.4. Obtaining supplies and procurement: This includes procurement activities, such as purchasing products. The tasks encompass choosing suppliers, deciding on order timelines and quantities, and coordinating product delivery. This is done to ensure that the right products are acquired on time and in sufficient amounts to meet the needs of various hospital service units.

Our hospital's procurement procedures align with the Prime Minister's Office Procurement Regulations, B.E. 2535, and the Drug and Non-Drug Supplies Management Regulations, B.E. 2557. Our procurement division functions independently, organized by product groups. For example, the pharmacy department is responsible for procuring both medicinal and non-medicinal supplies, as well as general medical materials. The general administration department oversees the acquisition of office supplies. The laboratory handles the purchase of autopsy materials, although certain items are shared

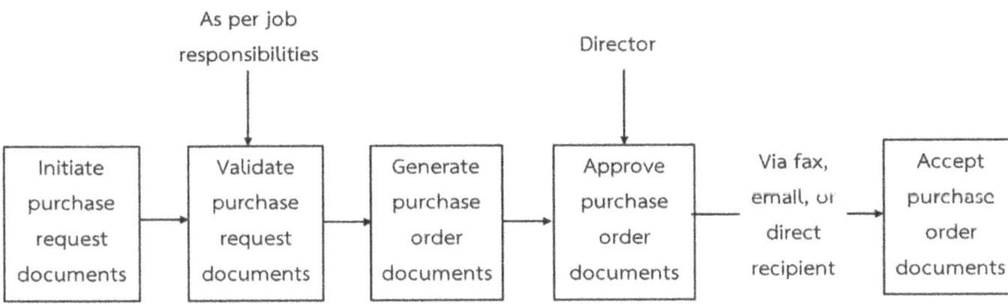

Figure 1.8. Workflow diagram of the hospital's product procurement process. (Kritchanchai & Srisakunwan, 2023a).

with the Subdistrict Health Promotion Hospital network. The pharmacy department takes care of procuring this group of products. Meanwhile, the dental unit manages the entire dental material procurement process.

For their procurement needs, community hospitals typically use two models: joint purchasing, which is facilitated by the provincial public health department, and general purchasing, which is carried out by the hospital itself. Here is a brief overview (Figure 1.8):

Joint purchasing	This involves ordering medicines and medical supplies that have a high usage rate, such as items for Non-Communicable Diseases (NCDs), as well as less frequently used items to benefit from economies of scale. Hospitals forward their demand for drugs and medical supplies to the provincial public health department, which then procures them at a median price and selects the seller accordingly.
General purchasing	The hospital engages in direct procurement, purchasing directly from sellers. Additionally, procurement is also carried out for the Subdistrict Health Promotion Hospital network.

To ensure adequate product availability for upcoming service needs, the hospital has an annual purchasing plan. For each procurement period, purchase orders are utilized as the primary mechanism.

Throughout the year, purchases are made and categorized by product group: medicines, non-medicinal supplies, medical materials, supplies, and equipment. These acquisitions are overseen by the respective department responsible for each product type. The quantities ordered are determined based on historical usage data, current inventory levels, and projected future needs. During potential disease outbreaks, which are often seasonal, the demand for drug reserves increases. The reorder point is reached when the stock of a product drops below the average monthly usage rate. At this point, we restock to an amount equivalent to 1.5–2 months of usage.

Once you have determined the quantity of products to order, the agency issues a purchase order and follows approval procedures. Each order must receive approval from the director. If approval cannot be secured in time, the hospital mitigates this by borrowing products from vendors in advance and issues the purchase order at a later date.

When a purchase order receives the director's approval, the agency primarily communicates this to vendors via fax, email, or phone. The principal vendors encompass the Government Pharmaceutical Organization, along with various private distributor companies. As of now, vendors do not have a system in place to provide advance notifications of product deliveries. Instead, a general delivery timeframe, typically around one month, is established.

The hospital not only procures drugs and medical supplies directly but also benefits from the National Health Security Office's drug reimbursement program. The program provides supplemental resources for drugs and medical supplies. The pharmacy department logs the usage of drugs and medical supplies acquired through the Prescription Drug and Medical Supplies Reimbursement Program. Upon receipt of these data, the National Health Security Office arranges for the compensation of the aforementioned items. On a case-by-case basis, the hospital may receive these drugs and medical supplies free of charge from the provincial health office, depending on various projects.

Simultaneously, the hospital serves a crucial role as a link, gathering the overall medicine and medical supply demands from the subdistrict health promotion hospitals within its network. It is the hospital's responsibility to issue all purchase orders.

Regarding the procurement of other product types, it has been observed that the department in charge of the respective product issues the purchase orders. They coordinate and follow up on orders directly with sellers. For instance, the general management departments handle the purchase of office supplies and equipment, among others.

Issues have been identified in the procurement process, mainly due to its time-consuming nature and the multiple procedures involved. Uncertainty in product delivery, especially for items in short supply, causes delays. Consequently, hospitals are forced to maintain larger reserves, which could potentially result in a lack of financial liquidity. This is particularly notable in the drug and medical supply group.

1.2.5. Estimating product demand (Forecasting): This task involves projecting future product demand across various service units. Advanced estimation serves as a planning tool for preparing products, personnel, or equipment. Any inaccuracies in these estimates can have a direct impact on cost factors such as storage, ordering, and transportation. Additionally, they could result in either a shortage or surplus of products, failing to meet service recipient needs, or leading to unnecessary waste due to product deterioration or expiration.

Most hospitals create their annual product usage estimates primarily for budgeting purposes. However, when it comes to estimating product usage for shorter periods such as quarterly or monthly, there is often a lack of specific action.

Nonetheless, replenishment strategies are coordinated between the service unit and the warehouse. A maximum quantity for each type of product is set, serving as a framework for each service unit's product list. This ensures that there are enough products to cover each product's disbursement cycle. For instance, if the disbursement cycle is one week, the maximum quantity stored would correspond to one week of usage. In the event that the service unit does not have enough stock items for a week, they will coordinate with neighboring units to borrow the necessary products. After receiving their disbursement in the next round, the service unit will then compensate the unit that provided the borrowed items. Alternatively, the service unit may request an emergency pick-up from the warehouse in case neighboring units face the same shortage issue.

Quantitative estimates are not often seen because the information system might not be equipped to gather and process balance data and product usage rates at an organizational level. As a result, most estimates tend to be qualitative.

1.2.6. Logistics management information system: This refers to the transmission and exchange of logistics information. Effective communication among different service units within the hospital, including with external stakeholders, is crucial. It significantly impacts decision-making, enabling faster and more efficient operations.

In the majority of hospitals, there are two primary categories of information technology in use: patient services information systems and warehouse management information systems. Here are the details:

Patient services	The primary information system for most patient services is the HOSxP program. Often, this is used in conjunction with the LIS program for the analysis of medical technology laboratory results. With the LIS program, analysis results can be directly transmitted to the HOSxP program, enabling doctors to make disease diagnoses more efficiently.
Warehouse management	The system's responsibility involves managing a medical supply warehouse, which includes both pharmaceuticals and non-drug medical supplies, such as dental and autopsy materials. Product distribution is regulated through the use of the INV DOS program or custom-developed software, in conjunction with product control cards. In addition, the warehouse department also handles office supplies, housekeeping, and kitchen supplies. Control over product distribution is maintained using hospital-developed software or standard programs, such as Microsoft Access.

Beyond the mentioned programs, the hospital is progressively integrating information technology into various tasks. For instance, the system has incorporated a digital X-ray system that can transmit data electronically, offering an advantage over the traditional film method.

1.2.7. Transportation and distribution of products to service units or patients: This activity involves the efficient transportation of products from the storage location to the point of demand, ensuring completeness, accuracy, perfect condition, and timely delivery.

Most hospitals handle two types of transportation: patient movement and goods movement. The details are as follows:

Patient movement	Patient movement pertains to patients who are present to receive services. If a patient can manage independently, they navigate themselves to respective service units. However, should a patient require assistance, a dedicated worker is assigned for patient aid and transportation across different service units.
Goods transportation	This involves the transportation of various items used within the hospital, from their storage or staging location to their point of usage.

Freight can be categorized into three types: delivery by the originating service unit, pickup by the destination service unit, and shared responsibilities. The details are as follows:

Delivery by the originating service unit	The service support unit acts as a leader in delivery, distributing sterile medical supplies to patient wards, dental rooms, and other units like laundry, ensuring provision of clean clothes.
Pick-up by the destination service unit	Service units retrieve the product from the delivery point and transport it to their respective areas. This includes receiving medicines and medical supplies as per doctor's prescriptions, and requisitioning supplies, equipment, and so forth.
Shared responsibilities	In a joint effort, service units and service support units carry out transportation operations. This could involve a ward collecting used clothes and delivering it to a central collection point, where the laundry unit would then collect and clean it. For waste management, the service unit is responsible for collecting waste from its area and delivering it to temporary collection points. Subsequently, the housekeeper from the waste unit collects and disposes of it in accordance with waste type regulations.

Table 1.2. Categories of goods transportation within the hospital.

Product	Responsible Person		Details
	Origin	Destination	
Patient	—	—	Stretcher or patient.
Food	•	—	The nutrition unit is responsible for the delivery and distribution of food to patients, as well as the collection of used food containers. Nurses occasionally perform random checks on patient meals to ensure accuracy.
Linen	•	—	The service unit gathers used linen and delivers it to the designated area. From there, the laundry unit takes over, ensuring the linen is properly cleaned and then returned to the service unit for afternoon pick-up.
Outpatient medicine	—	—	Medicine collected by the patient.
Inpatient medicine	—	•	The ward collects prescriptions, while the warehouse replenishes medicine supplies according to a schedule.
Medical materials	—	•	Service units collect items from the medical supplies warehouse at scheduled times.
Medical supplies	—	•	Service units collect items from the medical supplies warehouse at scheduled times.
Sterile medical supplies	—	•	Service units deliver used medical supplies with delivery slips and exchange them for sterile supplies at agreed intervals.
Waste	•	•	The service unit delivers waste to the designated garbage collection point. The housekeeper of the garbage unit comes to collect and dispose of the waste.

Note: • It is the transport operator; — not the transport operator.

As mentioned earlier, the majority of transportation patterns within hospitals are summarized in Table 1.2.

The frequency of transportation for goods varies depending on the product type. We determine this by estimating the total usage for each product type. For instance, you can consider the detailed example from a hospital, as shown in Table 1.3.

Table 1.3. Product disbursement frequency in a hospital.

Product	Disbursement Frequency
Outpatient medicine	• Dispensed daily from the medicine room for outpatients, inpatients, and accident and emergency patients. • Stockpile medicine for the accident and emergency room is dispensed daily outside of business hours for accident and emergency patients.
Inpatient medicine	• Prescription medicines are dispensed daily. • The service unit houses a stockpile of medicines, including life-saving drugs, cold medications, and blood pressure medicines. These can be replenished as they are used. • Saltwater reserves are maintained in the service unit and are replenished weekly.
Medical supplies	These are distributed on a weekly basis.
Medical materials	These are distributed on a weekly basis.
Patient food	We ensure the provision of three meals a day for patients.
Linen	The service team transports used laundry to designated rest areas, which are then collected by the laundry team twice daily—once in the morning and once in the afternoon. As for clean clothes, the service team will retrieve them in the afternoon.

1.3 Conclusion

Hospital logistics is the invisible framework that supports every aspect of patient care. This chapter explained how logistics connects facilities, people, and systems, ensuring that materials, information, and finances move seamlessly through the hospital network. By breaking down the hospital supply chain into nodes, links, and flows, readers gained a clear understanding of how medicines, equipment, and supplies reach the right place at the right time. The discussion highlighted the interconnectedness of logistics activities and emphasized that inefficiencies in one area can ripple across the entire system.

The lessons from this chapter demonstrate that logistics is not limited to transportation or storage but rather is an integrated system that impacts patient safety, treatment speed, and overall hospital efficiency. By mapping out the flows of materials and information, hospitals can identify duplication, delays, or unclear responsibilities. This systematic perspective empowers healthcare managers to redesign processes in ways that reduce waste and enhance the quality of service delivered to patients.

Chapter 2

Effective Inventory Management in Hospitals

This section covers node management within the inventory sector. The essence of inventory management is to maintain optimal stock levels through careful planning and control. To meet service requirements while keeping inventory costs low, inventory may be stored across various locations within the hospital, primarily at distribution holding and staging points. The distribution holding areas serve as the initial receiving areas for goods from suppliers. These are the areas where goods are held before they are dispatched to their points of use. On the other hand, the staging points are the areas where goods are held in anticipation of use. These include medicine rooms, wards, and operating rooms, where products are held before being distributed to patients. Regardless of product type, any item held in storage is considered inventory, and all inventory incurs administrative and holding costs.

Inventory management aims to achieve the following objectives:

1. Maintain sufficient stock levels to meet service requirements.
2. Minimize inventory investment to the lowest practical level.
3. Identify the optimal order quantity and reorder point.
4. Maintain liquidity by ensuring a swift product turnover rate.
5. Mitigate potential future uncertainties.
6. Prevent overstocking that could lead to insufficient storage space.

2.1 Types of Inventories in the Logistics System

There are five types of inventories in the logistics system:

1. **Cycle/Regular Stock**: This inventory supports cyclical demand during normal operations.
2. **Safety Stock**: This is a reserve inventory.
3. **Seasonal Stock**: These are products stored for seasonal demand.
4. **In-Transit Inventory**: These are goods at different stages of the transport route, from the factory to the customer.
5. **Other Stock**: This is additional stock for other reasons.

Often, an inventory control system separates products into ABC categories based on the product's value and usage.

Annual demand X cost per unit

- Category A products make up 20% of the item count, contributing to 80% of the total value.
- Category B products constitute 30% of the item count, equating to 15% of the total value.
- Category C products represent 50% of the item count but equate to only 5% of the total value.

To enhance our inventory management system, our primary focus should be on managing Category A inventory, given its high value. This approach could potentially have a significant impact on reducing hospital costs.

Inventory management definitions

- **Order Quantity (Q)**: The quantity of an order.
- **Reorder Point (ROP)**: The inventory level that triggers a new order.
- **Usage Rate**: The rate at which inventory is used.
- **Average Inventory**: The average inventory level, calculated as Q/2.
- **Supplier Lead Time**: The duration between placing an order and receiving the product.
- **Holding (Carrying) Costs**: The costs associated with storing a product, such as sunk costs and interest on storage and handling, typically calculated as 20–30% of the product's value.

- **Ordering Costs**: The costs incurred during the ordering process, which include time, paperwork expenses, and communication.
- **Shortage Costs**: Costs related to product shortages.

To illustrate the relationship between three terms, Figure 2.1 presents the inventory level and duration of a simple stock as an example.

The inventory management approach commonly used in hospitals is the Economic Order Quantity (EOQ), also known as the Q-system.

This system provides an economical ordering estimate by primarily focusing on holding (Carrying) costs and ordering costs (Figure 2.2). This graph illustrates that if we place a large order at once, the holding cost will increase, but the ordering cost will decrease. On the other hand, placing smaller, more frequent orders will increase procurement costs but lower holding costs. Therefore, it is essential to discover the optimal Order Quantity Q* or EOQ point to minimize the total cost.

The formula to calculate this is

$$\text{EOQ} = \text{Q}^* = \sqrt{\frac{2\,\text{DS}}{\text{H}}}.$$

In this formula,

- EOQ, Q* represent the most economical order quantity,
- D stands for Demand per cycle time,

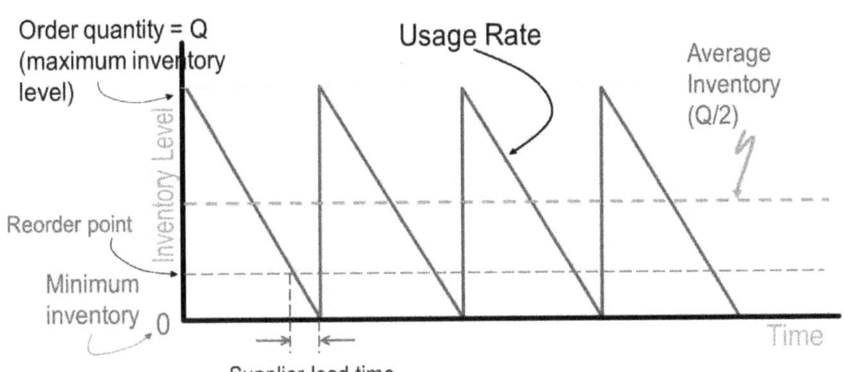

Figure 2.1. A graph demonstrating the relationship between inventory levels and duration.
Source: Adapted from Operations management: Sustainability and supply chain management (13th ed.), by J. Heizer, B. Render, and C. Munson, 2020, Pearson.

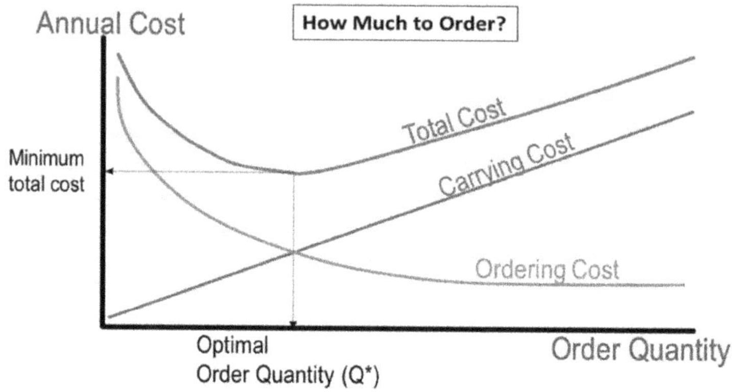

Figure 2.2. A graph displaying the correlation between total cost and order quantity.
Source: Adapted from Supply chain management: Strategy, planning, and operation (6th ed.), by S. Chopra and P. Meindl, 2016, Pearson.

- H represents the holding/carrying cost per unit per cycle time, and
- S is the ordering cost per order.

This allows us to determine the following:

- the number of orders per cycle time $N = \frac{D}{Q*}$,
- the time between orders $T = \frac{\text{Working day}}{N}$, and
- the total cost

$$TC = \text{Ordering cost} + \text{Carrying cost} = \frac{D}{Q}S + \frac{Q}{2}H.$$

2.2 Case Study of Inventory Management Problem in a Hospital

Effective inventory management is a key factor in controlling hospital management costs. Many hospitals, regardless of size, prioritize inventory management, encompassing the processes of ordering, forecasting, storage, and distribution. Today, advances in logistics and technology, including data science and artificial intelligence (AI), have led to improved forecasting and inventory management systems. These AI models help predict product demand with greater accuracy, enhancing inventory management efficiency, reducing lead times and reorder points, and lowering inventory levels. This results in cost savings, less waste from expired medications, and fewer drug shortages.

Consider the following example: A large hospital has implemented a volume prediction system for inventory management, by utilizing AI technology over a 5G network, focusing on the following:

- The process of purchasing and importing medication and medical supplies is being studied. This covers everything, from placing orders with distributors or suppliers to receiving the medication in the central drug warehouse.
  - The secondary data sourced from hospital databases includes the following:
    1. **Purchase orders**: This includes information about the central drug warehouse's procurement of drugs and medical supplies.
    2. **Product receipts**: Information concerning the reception of medicines and medical supplies from the central drug warehouse.
    3. **Stock information**: Details regarding the quantity of drugs and medical supplies stored within the central drug warehouse.
    4. **Dispensation**: Information about drug dispensing.

In developing a policy for managing these medicines and medical supplies, Consideration is given to the large number of items involved Consequently, the focus on the group of drugs and medical supplies with the highest usage (dispensing) value. We have selected items from various groups for this purpose. Note that the aforementioned list of medical supplies does not include those pro-duced by the hospital itself.

2.2.1 *An assessment of the current ordering and inventory management processes*

Our hospital uses the SAP system for drug and medical supply inventory management. This Enterprise Resource Planning (ERP) system helps streamline the disbursement, ordering, and replenishment of drugs and medical supplies according to demand. It calculates the demand at each service point and the central drug warehouse to process orders through SAP's MRP (Material Requirement Planning) module. The central drug warehouse then undertakes the task of picking up and delivering medicines and medical supplies to various service points. This ensures a smooth flow of supplies, preventing shortages and overstocking. Recently, we have incorporated new technology into our system: we are using artificial intelligence to help forecast the demand for drugs and medical supplies. This means we can manage our inventory even more effectively. Our study aimed to develop a new inventory management policy that uses artificial intelligence to handle large amounts of data, replacing the previous system. This use of AI will enhance the hospital's current work systems, making them more accurate and efficient. Our investigation focused on the lot sizing policy. We looked at the relationship between demand patterns from all 52 samples of drugs and medical supplies with the highest usage value and the order quantity, usage rate, and number of medical supplies in stock. These data will serve as a case study for the entire sample group. The order will be determined according to the most economical order quantity (Economic Order Quantity: EOQ).

2.2.2 *Procedures and tools used for calculation*

During the ABC and FSN analysis grouping, we use mathematical tools to understand the demand and distribution of drugs and medical supplies. Each tool serves a unique purpose:

1. We use the ABC classification principle for grouping. Here, medicines and medical supplies are divided into three categories based on their usage value: high (A), medium (B), and low (C). The division proportions are shown in Table 2.1.
2. The turnover ratio, or proportion of turnover, is a methodology used in FSN analysis to understand the movement of drugs and medical supplies. This is done by assessing the frequency of imports to the central warehouse.

   - F (Fast) refers to frequent movement, involving the import of drugs or medical supplies more than twice a month.
   - S (Slow) indicates less frequent movement, with imports happening approximately twice a month.

- N (Non-moving) refers to minimal or no movement, with imports occurring less frequently than once every two months.

To maximize the use of available data, we have applied these calculations across the data set, leading us to the following additional criteria for FSN analysis grouping:

- F category drugs or medical supplies have a turnover of more than four cycles per month (turnover ratio ≥ 52 cycles per year).
- S category items have a turnover of approximately two cycles per month (turnover ratio 26–51 cycles per year).
- N category items have a turnover of less than two cycles per month (turnover ratio < 26 cycles per year).

3. Order up to level is a tool that sets order levels to facilitate decision-making. It is calculated using the formula

$$S = \mu + z \times \sigma$$

where

- S represents the maximum stock level,
- μ indicates the average demand within the ordering cycle, including delivery lead time plus one day,
- z is the standard value used to determine the service level (for instance, z-scores at service levels of 98%, 95%, and 90%), and
- σ is the standard deviation of demand within the order cycle, including delivery lead time plus one day.

4. The Shapiro–Wilk test is a method used to classify distribution patterns, with a focus on analyzing data distributions.
5. Linear regression, or R-squared, is a tool used to recognize and take into account demand trends.

Table 2.1. Classification proportions based on the usage value percentage of drugs and medical supplies, using the ABC classification principle.

Group of Medicines and Medical Supplies	Percentage of Value in Medicines and Medical Supplies	Percentage of Count in Medicine and Medical Supplies (%)
A	First 70–80% of usage value	10–15
B	Next 15–20% of usage value	30–40
C	Final 5–10% of usage value	50–60

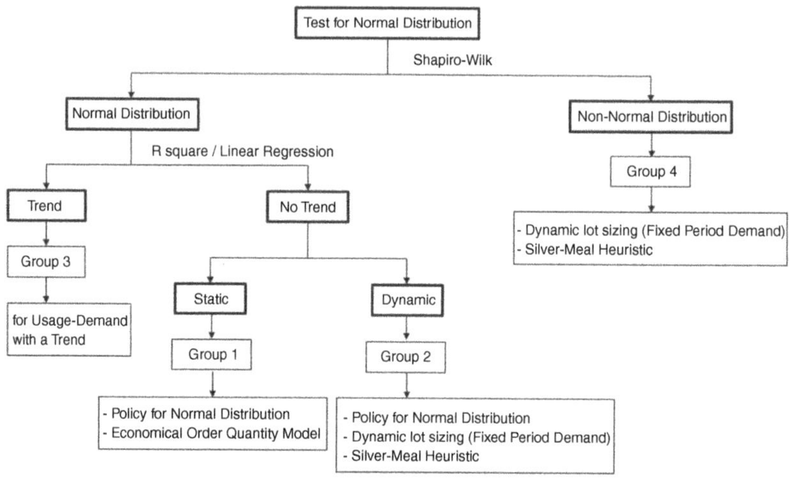

Figure 2.3. Steps for needs analysis to categorize drugs and medical supplies.

6. Peterson–Silver Law: A tool utilized for assessing demand fluctuation. It aids in determining whether a fixed or variable order size is most suitable.

Inventory models are as follows:

1. Economic Order Quantity (EOQ) model,
2. Fixed period demand,
3. Silver–Meal heuristic method.

A review of the literature on the development of inventory management in hospitals revealed that the characteristics of drug and medical supply demand can be categorized into four types (Figure 2.3):

1. Normal distribution, no trend, constant demand.
2. Normal distribution, no trend, non-constant demand.
3. Normal distribution with a trend.
4. Non-normal distribution.

2.2.3 *Case Study: Four Types of Demand Patterns*

2.2.3.1 *Type I: Normal distribution, no trend, constant demand*

We observe a normal distribution with no apparent trend and a steady demand. Our inventory management policy is outlined as follows:

2.2.3.1.1 When delivery times are unpredictable, we calculate new order points using this formula

$$\text{ROP} = \bar{d} \times \bar{L} + z\sqrt{\bar{d}^2\sigma_L^2}.$$

In this formula, ROP is the new order point:

- $\bar{d}$ is the average demand,
- L is the average delivery time,
- z is a standard value or score, and
- σ_L is the standard deviation of delivery time.

2.2.3.1.2 When delivery times are reliable, we use a simpler formula for new order points

$$\text{ROP} = \bar{d} \times L,$$

where ROP is the new order point,

- $\bar{d}$ is the average demand and
- L is the delivery time.

After determining a new order point, we compare vendor delivery times to the central drug warehouse. We then adjust our inventory policy as needed, based on how the drugs and medical supplies behave.

We use a normal distribution policy (s,S):

$$S = M\frac{\mu_{\text{week}}}{n} + k + s.$$

In this formula, S is the maximum inventory level of the product (unit),

- μ_{week} is the average demand per week (unit),
- M is the storage day (day),
- n is the service time per week (days), and
- k is the quantity of special demand that is known first and is the point at which new orders are made.

We also use a policy based on the economic ordering (EOQ) model (s,Q):

$$Q = \sqrt{\frac{2AD}{h}}.$$

In this formula, Q is the quantity ordered,

- D is the demand during the period (unit).
- A is the cost of purchasing per purchase (unit) and
- h is the annual inventory-keeping cost (Baht/unit/year).

2.2.3.2 *Type II: Normal distribution, no trend, non-constant demand*

In a scenario of normal distribution with no trend and non-constant demand, the following inventory management policy applies.

2.2.3.2.1 For unstable delivery times where the supplier fails to deliver on schedule, the formula to calculate new order points is

$$\text{ROP} = \bar{d} \times \bar{L} + z\sqrt{\bar{L}\sigma_d^2 + \bar{d}^2\sigma_L^2}.$$

In this equation, ROP represents the new order point. Further variables are

- d = average demand, (unit)
- L = average delivery time, (unit)
- z = standard value or score, (unit)
- σ_d = standard deviation of demand, (unit) and
- σ_L = standard deviation of delivery time.

2.2.3.2.2 In instances where the supplier delivers on schedule, the formula for calculating new order points is

$$\text{ROP} = \bar{d} \times L + z\sqrt{\bar{L}\sigma_d^2},$$

where ROP is the new order point,

- d = average demand, (unit)
- L = delivery time, (unit)
- z = standard value or score, and
- σ_d = standard deviation of demand (unit).

After determining a new order point, an analysis is conducted considering the supplier's delivery time to the central drug warehouse. The inventory policy is then adapted according to the behavior of drugs and medical supplies (item 2) as needed.

The normal distribution policy (s,S) is

$$S = M\frac{\mu_{\text{week}}}{n} + k + s,$$

where S is the maximum inventory level of the product (unit),

- μ_{week} = average demand per week (unit),
- M = storage day (day),
- n = service time per week (days),
- k = quantity of special demand that is known first, and
- s = point at which new orders are made.

Also, the dynamic lot sizing (Fixed Period Demand) where

- Q = average weekly demand * 4
  - Here, Q represents the order quantity.

Lastly, the silver–meal heuristic:

$$C_T = \frac{C_p + \sum_{i=1}^{T}(i-1)r_i C_h}{i},$$

where C_T = average cost of the order size,

- C_p = Ordering cost, (unit)
- C_h = Cost of holding inventory (Holding cost)
- i = preliminary procurement period, and (unit)
- r = product demand in perted: (iEI)

2.2.3.3 *Type III: Normal distribution with a trend*

We are applying a conventional inventory management model and policy that adheres to a normal distribution and trend. The policy for anticipated demand (s,Q) is as follows:

$$Q = \int_{t=a}^{t=b} f(d_t)dt + k,$$

where Q is the quantity to be ordered,

- k: Known special demand volume,
- A: Inventory collection commencement date, and
- B: Inventory collection completion date.

2.2.3.4 *Type IV: Normal distribution, no trend, constant demand*

In case of, the distribution does not follow a normal pattern. We can proceed by implementing the inventory management model and policy in the following ways.

2.2.3.4.1 Method to determine new order points for variable delivery times

This is relevant when a merchant is unable to ensure timely product delivery.

$$\text{ROP} = \bar{d} \times \bar{L} + z\sqrt{\bar{L}\sigma_d^2 + \bar{d}^2\sigma_L^2},$$

where ROP is the new order point,

- d: average demand,
- L: average delivery time,
- z: standard score,
- σ_d: standard deviation of demand (unit), and
- σ_L: standard deviation of delivery time (unit).

2.2.3.4.2 Method for determining new order points in fixed delivery time scenarios

This applies when a merchant delivers a product on time:

$$\text{ROP} = \bar{d} \times L + z\sqrt{\bar{L}\sigma_d^2},$$

where ROP is the new order point,

- d: average demand, (unit)
- L: delivery time, (unit)
- z: standard score, and
- σ_d: standard deviation of demand. (unit)

Once a new order point is determined, we analyze it based on the vendor's delivery time to the central drug warehouse. We consider the inventory policy appropriate based on the behavior of drugs and medical supplies in item 4.

Dynamic Lot Sizing (Fixed Period Demand):

- Q = average weekly demand ** 4
  - Q: order quantity (unit)

Silver–Meal Heuristic:

$$C_T = \frac{C_p + \sum_{i=1}^{T} (i-1) r_i C_h}{i},$$

where C_T is the average cost of the order size, (unit)

- C_p: ordering cost, (unit)
- Cost of holding inventory (holding cost),

Table 2.2. A breakdown of drug inventory management strategies based on demand characteristics.

Group	Demand Characteristics	Management Strategy Based on Literature Review
1	Demand with a normal distribution, no stable trend	(s,S) Policy for normal distribution of drug demand (s,Q) Policy for stable drug demand, orders in package size (s,Q) Policy using EOQ values
2	Demand with a normal distribution, no trend in variance	(s,S) Policy for normal distribution of drug demand (s,Q) Policy for variable drug demand, orders in package size Silver Meal
3	Likely demand with a normal distribution	(s,Q) Policy
4	Non-normal distribution of demand	Silver Meal
—	Applicable to all the above scenarios	(s,Q) Policy, Maximum inventory replenishment (Order up to Level)

Note: Table 2.2 illustrates inventory management strategies in hospitals.

Source: Adapted from "Developing inventory management in hospital" by Kritchanchai, D. & Meesamut, W. (2015). *International Journal of Supply Chain Management*, 4(2), 11–19.

The ABC analysis classifies inventory into three categories (A,B, and C) based on demand volume, while the FSN analysis categorizes items into three level cording to turnover rate. Their integration forms nine groups in the ABC-FSN matrix, detailed in Table 2.3 and illustrated in Table 2.4.

- i: preliminary procurement period (unit), and
- r: product demand. (unit)

2.2.4 *The process for categorizing drug and medical supply list using ABCFSN Analysis*

The principles can be outlined as follows:

2.2.4.1 *Start with the categorization of drugs and medical supplies according to the ABC classification principle*

2.2.4.1.1 Gather historical data on the quantity of medicine dispensed at every clinic from January 2020 to June 2021, along with the selling price for each drug item.
2.2.4.1.2 Sort the list of medicines based on their usage value, which is calculated as the quantity times the selling price, in descending order.
2.2.4.1.3 Calculate the percentage value of total drug use from the total drug value.
2.2.4.1.4 Use the ABC product grouping ratio (80:15:5) to calculate the total drug value and determine the value of drugs and medical supplies in each group (A, B, and C).
2.2.4.1.5 Compare the usage value of each group (A, B, and C) with the cumulative usage value in descending order to determine the number of drug items in each group.
2.2.4.1.6 From the number of drug items in each group found in Step 1.5, calculate the percentage based on the value of the drugs allocated to each group.
2.2.4.1.7 Repeat Steps 2.2.4.1.1–2.2.4.1.6 for medical supplies

2.2.4.2 *Demand-based classification using FSN principles*

The turnover ratio of medicines and medical supplies is a crucial measure of inventory management efficiency. This can be calculated

Table 2.3. Breakdown of the nine product groups in the ABC-FSN matrix analysis.

Group	Details	Label
1	High-use, high-turnover medicines and medical supplies	AF
2	High-use, moderate-turnover medicines and medical supplies	AS
3	High-use, low-turnover medicines and medical supplies	AN
4	Medium-use, high-turnover medicines and medical supplies	BF
5	Medium-use, moderate-turnover medicines and medical supplies	BS
6	Medium-use, low-turnover medicines and medical supplies	BN
7	Low-use, high-turnover medicines and medical supplies	CF
8	Low-use, moderate-turnover medicines and medical supplies	CS
9	Low-use, low-turnover medicines and medical supplies	CN

Table 2.4. Categorization by demand volume and drug movement (ABC-FSN Matrix).

Drug Group	F	S	N
A	AF	AS	AN
B	BF	BS	BN
C	CF	CS	CN

by dividing the volume of drugs and medical supplies by the average inventory quantity. Medicines and medical supplies can then be categorized according to their turnover rates, which can be tailored to suit the needs of the central medicine warehouse in monitoring inventory management efficiency. These groups include F (Fast moving), S (Slow moving), and N (Non moving). The turnover rate calculation typically utilizes average daily inventory data. However, as this data is not currently available, we will use the month-end inventory data in this report as an initial measure.

Turnover rate t is equal to total usage of that inventory/average inventory quantity of that inventory,

$$\text{Turnover Ratio} = \frac{\text{total usage of that inventory (unit)}}{\text{average inventory quantity of that inventory (unit)}}.$$

2.2.4.3 *Product type analysis using ABC-FSN matrix analysis*

This analysis focuses on the categorization of drugs and medical supplies. It uses the ABC analysis to sort items based on demand quantity and the FSN analysis to group them by turnover rate. These two analyses together form a metric that aids in determining quantity and the best ordering strategy for medications and medical supplies.

2.2.4.3.1 The analysis of the maximum inventory quantity (order up to level)

The demand delivery lead time between the hospital and the supplier was analyzed using the dataset. A majority of the drugs and medical supplies fall under Group A, which represents high usage value, as shown in Table 2.3.

However, to ensure comprehensive analysis, we have included items outside Group A as well. This includes all categories of drugs and medical supplies available in the hospital, even those classified by importance, such as life-saving or Group V. When inventory levels reach the reorder point, the central drug warehouse can place an order to prevent shortages.

The method for determining the maximum inventory quantity (order up to level) is suitable for managing the central drug warehouse in the hospital. It ensures a continuous supply of medical items without maintaining an excessive inventory. The guidelines are as follows:

- Group A and life-saving items will be replenished at least once a week.
- Group B items are replenished every 2 weeks.
- Group C items will be replenished monthly. If the items are large, they will be replenished weekly.

The formula for determining the maximum inventory quantity corresponds to with Tables 2.5 and 2.6:

$$S = \mu + z \times \sigma,$$

where

- S is the maximum stock level,
- μ is the average demand during the ordering cycle, plus lead time for delivery, plus one day unit,
- z is a standard value to determine the service level (for service levels of 98%, 95%, and 90%), and
- σ is the standard deviation of demand in the order cycle plus delivery lead time plus one day (unit).

Additionally, we have a formula to calculate the order point for fluctuating demand with a fixed delivery time:

$$\text{ROP} = dL + z\sqrt{\bar{L}\sigma_d^2}.$$

Each component corresponds to the following:

- ROP is the new order point unit,
- dL is the daily demand, which is equal to the number of delivery days unit,
- z is a standard value (2.05, 1.65, and 1.28 for service levels of 98%, 95%, and 90%, respectively), and
- σ_d is the standard deviation of demand.

The table above provides data on the average daily demand, standard deviation of average daily demand, and average delivery time. For our analysis, we have used the formula for calculating the maximum inventory quantity as follows:

$$S = \mu + z \times \sigma,$$

where

- S stands for the maximum stock level unit,
- μ represents the average demand in the order and delivery lead time plus one day unit,
- z is the standard value for determining the service level (z-score at service level of 98%, 95%, 90%), and
- σ is the standard deviation of demand in the order cycle and delivery lead time plus one day.

2.2.4.3.2 The analysis of ordering costs and inventory storage costs (holding costs)

Inventory holding costs can be described as:

$$\text{Inventory holding cost} = \text{Inventory value} \times (\beta + i).$$

The inventory value from the central drug and medical supply warehouse is derived from calculations and cost data analysis for 16 months, from January 2020 to June 2021.

Table 2.5. The cost components of holding goods.

Average Costs	Percent[1] (%)	B
1. Tax	0.50	0.50
2. Depreciation	8.25	8.25
3. Deteriorated Goods	10.00	0.00995[2]
4. Insurance	0.25	0.25
Total	19	9.00995

Average holding costs (β) represent the average of various product ownership-related expenses, such as taxes, damages, depreciation, costs of deteriorated products, and insurance costs.

The assumption is that the average cost of holding goods, or β, was previously a constant value of β equal to 19%,[1] which consists of the components as shown in Table 2.5.

The interest rate (i) represents the opportunity cost of holding goods. It is based on the average interest rate for prime customers (Minimum Lending Rate: MLR), as it is a suitable rate to represent the real costs for Thai entrepreneurs. Currently, the interest rate is 5.25% (2022 data) as shown in Table 2.5. Therefore, the cost of holding goods is calculated as follows:

$$\begin{aligned}\text{Product holding cost} &= \text{Inventory value} \times (9.00995 + 5.25)\\ &= \text{Inventory value} \times (14.25995).\end{aligned}$$

Note: The sum of $\beta + i$ equals 14.25%.

2.2.4.4 *The design and development of a dashboard in the dimension of inventory management at the drug/medical supply warehouse level produced the following results*

The report in Figure 2.4 shows the inventory management results at the drug/ medical supply warehouse level consists of 6 pages which contain the following details: The first table explains the ABC method, which groups products by demand value (usage × price) to optimize inventory, and the FSN method, which classifies items by

[1] Alford–Bangs Production Handbook Formula 1975.
[2] Average data of obsolete goods from sample hospitals in 2020 and 2021.

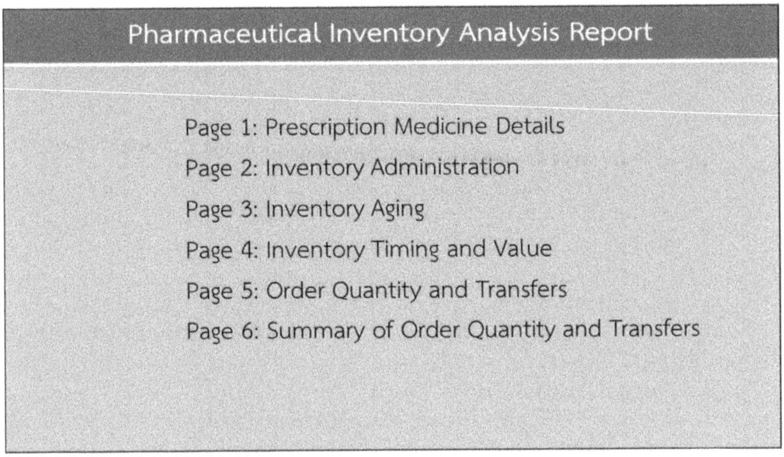

Figure 2.4. Pharmaceutical inventory analysis report.
Note: The term "capital investment/value" indicates the value obtained from the selling price, not the cost, when shown as a financial figure.

turnover rate (Fast, Slow, Non-moving) to prioritize stock efficiently. Tables 2.7–2.8 provide an overview of key metrics (e.g., purchase orders, costs, and lead times) alongside graphical data, including medical supply transfers to warehouses. Tables 2.9–2.10 focuses on aging inventory performance, covering service life, medication room codes, expiration tracking, and shortage warnings. Finally, Tables 2.11–2.12 details order quantities and transfers, with filters to summarize total quantities and withdrawal trends for analysis.

Each report page shows the product groupings, arranged by the ABC and FSN methods, providing the details in Table 2.6.

Table 2.6. KPI details.

KPI	Details
ABC	The thought processes of Group ABC can be outlined as follows: 1. Determine the average demand based on the past 90 days and gather information on the value or selling price of each drug item. 2. Organize the list of medicines based on their usage value in descending order (Usage value = Demand × Selling price). 3. Compute the percentage value of total drug usage from the total drug value.

Table 2.6. (*Continued*)

KPI	Details
	4. Use the ABC product grouping proportion (80:15:5) on the total drug value, and multiply these proportions to ascertain the value of drugs/medical supplies in each group A, B, and C. 5. Use the drug usage values for each group A, B, and C and compare the sum of the drug usage values arranged by value from highest to lowest. This helps identify the number of drug items in each group A, B, and C. 6. Utilize the number of drug items in each group obtained from Step 5 to calculate the percentage of the value of drugs allocated to each group.
FSN	Let us group FSN using these thought processes: The turnover rate is calculated as follows: $\text{Turnover}_{\text{rate}} = \frac{\text{Sum of demand (quantity withdrawn) in the past 90 days}}{\text{Average on hand inventory in the same period}},$ where • **Sum of demand (quantity withdrawn) in the past 90 days** refers to the total demand values (quantity withdrawn) for each drug over the past 90 days, and • **Average on-hand inventory in the same period** denotes the average daily on-hand value during this 90-day period. Based on the results, the categories can be defined as follows: ◇ F category items have at least 13 turnovers per quarter. ◇ S category items have a minimum of 6 turnovers per quarter. ◇ N category items have fewer than 6 turnovers per quarter.

2.2.4.4.1 Page 1: Purchasing metrics overview

This section outlines key purchasing metrics and options, including order status, warehouse, and date range. Core KPIs cover the number of purchase orders, total order value, ordering costs, and average lead time. Graphs and tables illustrate purchasing trends, order statistics, and vendor-specific data. Outline as follows:

- **Number of PO**: Total number of purchase orders.
- **Order value**: Total monetary value of all orders.

Table 2.7. Description of purchasing KPIs and information details.

KPI	Details
1. Overview information	• **Number of purchase orders**: This is the count of POs during the selected period. • **Number of medicines/medical supplies**: This is counted from the items in the PO sheet during the selected period. • **Value of ordering drugs/medical supplies**: This is the total value of orders for drugs/medical supplies during the selected period. • **Ordering costs**: This is calculated by multiplying the ordering cost per SKU by the number of times ordering: — Ordering cost per SKU of medicine at 141.65 baht. — Ordering cost per SKU of medical supplies at 157.12 baht • **Average Lead Time**: This is the average waiting time (from the order date until the delivery date) of each supplier during the selected period.
2. Graph showing purchasing value (baht)	This graph displays the total value of purchases for a selected period. It can be filtered by day, month, or year to view past statistics and trends.
3. Graph showing the number of purchase orders	This graph displays the total number of purchase orders for a selected period, which can be filtered by day, month, or year to view past statistics and trends.
4. Table showing orders for medicines and medical supplies (according to the list)	Displays the following information: — Drug/medical supply code — Name of medicine/medical supplies — ABC/FSN grouping — Material Group (#) — Number of purchase orders (#) — Order value (baht) — Lead Time (days)

- **Ordering costs**: Calculated as Baht/medicine SKU × number of orders.
- **Average lead time**: Number of days from order placement to delivery.

Table 2.7. (*Continued*)

KPI	Details
5. Table showing orders for drugs and medical supplies (according to vendor)	Displays the following information: — Vendor code — Number of purchase orders (#) — Order value (baht) — Percentage of purchase order value — Lead Time (days)
6. Table showing total details of the order	Displays the following information: — Purchase order code — Order date — Date of receipt — Drug/medical supply code — Name of medicine/medical supply — Vendor code — Purchasing status — Order value (baht) — Purchase amount (baht) — Number of shipments (#) — Lead Time (days) — Proportion of purchasing value
7. Graph showing the proportion of medicine items that have free gifts	This graph shows the number of medicines with and without free gifts.
8. Graph showing purchase quantity and percentage of free gifts (according to the list)	— The X-axis represents the time period in months. — The Y-axis depicts the quantity (axis 1). — The percentage of bonus is shown on axis 2.
9. Table showing the list of medicines/ medical supplies that have free gifts	Displays the following information: — Vendor code — Drug/medical supply code — Name of medicine/medical supply — Last order date — Purchase quantity (#/baht) — Free quantity — Order value (baht)

Table 2.8. Description of warehouse KPIs and information details.

KPI	Details
1. Overview Information	This section provides details about: — The number of medicine stocks (count) — The number of different medicines (in the medicine list) — The quantity of medical supplies (items)
2. Medicine and Medical Supplies Transfer Information (according to the medicine warehouse)	This section displays: — The code for the medicine room — The name of the medicine room — The quantity of items — The transfer value (baht),
3. Medicine and Medical Supplies Transfer Information	This section presents: — The code for the medicine room — The codes for the drugs and medical supplies — The names of medicines and medical supplies — ABC — FSN — Material Group — Service Level — The transfer value (baht),

2.2.4.4.2 Page 2: Warehouse management overview

This page presents a summary of warehouse operations, including current stock levels, transfer records between medicine rooms, and detailed item information. Filters are available to refine data by warehouse, material group, or date range. Additional vendor-related metrics are also included to enhance supplier analysis:

- **Vendor code**: Identifies suppliers and indicates order frequency.
- **Order value**: Reflects spending distribution across vendors.
- **Lead time**: Measures delivery speed by vendor.

2.2.4.4.3 Page 3: Aging inventory analysis

This section focuses on inventory aging, grouping items by their remaining lifespan. It summarizes usable life and inventory value and

Table 2.9. Description of aging inventory and information details.

Filter ◇ Estimated lifespan (1 year, 3 months, 6 months, more than 1 year, or expired)	
1. Aging Inventory	The information is structured into three distinct subsections as follows: 1. Overview of Service Life: — Remaining Useful Life (date) — Quantity (items) — Inventory Value (baht)
	2. Medication Room Codes: — Medication Room Code — Quantity (items) — Inventory Quantity (#) — Inventory Value (baht)
	3. Detailed Service Life Information: — Medication Room Code — Names of Medications and Medical Supplies — Expiration Date — Unit — Inventory Quantity (#) — Inventory Value (baht)
2. Table Displaying Drug Inventory – Warning of Potential Shortages	This is an informational display: — Code for Medicine Warehouse — Codes for Drugs and Medical Supplies — Names of Medicines and Medical Supplies — Inventory Quantity (#) — Average Daily Transfers — Remaining Supply (in days)

provides detailed expiration data. It also identifies potential shortages by displaying current stock levels and average daily transfers. Outline as follows:

- **Remaining useful life**: For example, expiration within 3 months.
- **Inventory value**: Stock volume and respective value.
- **Expiration dates**: Item-level expiry details.

Table 2.10. Description of inventory KPIs and information details.

KPI	Details
1. Introductory Information	This is a display of information: • Number of medicines (items). • Value of drug inventory (in baht) = Quantity on hand × Selling price per unit. • Number of medical supplies (items). • Value of medical supplies inventory (in baht) = Quantity on hand × Selling price per unit. • Average inventory period (in days) = Average inventory for 28 days/Average demand for 28 days. • The average inventory period does not include psychoactive substances, narcotic drugs, and chemicals. • Inventory value (in baht) = Value of medicines/ medical supplies inventory (in baht) × Holding cost rate = 14.25% (per year).
2. Graph Depicting Inventory Value (in Baht)	The X-axis represents the timeline (months). The Y-axis denotes the value of the inventory (baht).
3. Graph Illustrating Average Inventory Duration (in Days)	The X-axis still represents the timeline, in months. The Y-axis, this time, represents the average inventory period (days).
4. Detailed Table Presentation (Relevant to the Medicine Room)	The following details are displayed: — Code for the medicine room — Name of the medicine room — Quantity of items (#) — Average inventory period (days) — Value of inventory (baht) — Value of inventory (baht)

(*Continued*)

Table 2.10. (*Continued*)

KPI	Details
5. Detailed Table Presentation (Pertinent to the List)	The following information is displayed: — Code for the medicine room — Codes for drugs and medical supplies — Names of the medicines and medical supplies — ABC — FSN — Material Group — Average inventory period (days) — Value of inventory (baht) — Value of inventory (baht)

Table 2.11. Description of order and withdrawal KPIs and information details.

KPI	Details
1. Numerical data	This represents the quantity of medicines and medical supplies
2. Table showing detailed information (Explanation according to the Excel table above)	This includes information on the following: — Medicine warehouse — Drug/medical supply code — Name of medicine/medical supply — Material Group — ABC/FSN — Lead Time (unit) — Service Level — Average daily transfers (#) — Current Fixed Lot Size (#) — Suggested Fixed Lot Size (#) — Percentage Difference in Fixed Lot Size — Average Daily Demand (unit) — SAP Reorder Point (ROP) — Suggested ROP — SAP Safety Stock (#) — Suggested Safety Stock (#) — Purchase order quantity in the past 90 days (#) — Order quantity (#) — Surplus quantity (#)

Table 2.11. (*Continued*)

KPI	Details
3. Inventory Days efficiency comparison table (Calculation formula according to D1)	This table displays information on the following: — Medicine warehouse Drug/medical supply code — Name of medicine/medical supplies — Material Group — ABC/FSN — Current Fixed Lot Size (#) — Suggested Fixed Lot Size (#) — Order Up To Level
4. Table comparing average daily Inventory Cost efficiency (Calculation formula according to D2)	This table displays information on the following: — Medicine warehouse — Drug/medical supply code — Name of medicine/medical supplies — Material Group — ABC/FSN — Current Fixed Lot Size (#) — Suggested Fixed Lot Size (#) — Order Up To Level

2.2.4.4.4 Page 4: Inventory performance report

This report summarizes inventory value, average inventory holding period, and associated holding costs. Visual elements include charts for stock value and duration, while tables provide item-level or medicine room-level breakdowns. Outline as follows:

- **Inventory value**: Calculated as Quantity × Selling Price.
- **Holding cost**: Based on a 14.25% annual rate.
- **Average inventory period**: Number of days inventory is held.

2.2.4.4.5 Page 5: Order and Withdrawal Analysis

This section reviews order quantities and transfer withdrawals, offering item-level tables and comparisons of current versus suggested lot sizes. Graphs illustrate differences in holding costs and coverage days under various ordering approaches. Outline as follows:

Table 2.12. Description of inventory efficiency KPIs and information details.

KPI	Details
1. Overview information	Please refer to the following information: — Total count of medicines/medical supplies. — Detailed list of medicines/medical supplies that have been withdrawn. — Comprehensive list of medicines/medical supplies still in circulation.
2. Comparison graph of Inventory Holding Cost (drugs and medical supplies)	— The X-axis represents three different methods of order quantity calculation: Fixed lot size, Suggested Fixed Lot Size, and Order up to Level. — The Y-axis displays the corresponding cost in baht.
3. Inventory day comparison graph (number of days that products are sufficient for use according to transfer statistics) (drugs and medical supplies)	— The X-axis illustrates three methods of order quantity calculation: Fixed lot size, Suggested Fixed Lot Size, and Order up to Level. — The Y-axis indicates the number of days.

- **Current and suggested lot size**: Recommendations for adjustment.
- **Reorder points (ROP)**: SAP settings compared with recommended levels.
- **Safety stock**: Actual versus ideal buffer levels.

2.2.4.5.6 Page 6: Inventory Efficiency Comparison

This page evaluates inventory performance through cost and coverage comparisons, focusing on optimized ordering strategies such as fixed lot sizes and suggested adjustments. Chart axes represent:

- **X-axis**: Ordering methods (e.g., Fixed Lot Size and Order-Up-To Level).
- **Y-axis**: Costs or inventory coverage in days.

2.3 Conclusion

Inventory management is a critical challenge in hospitals, where balancing cost efficiency with uninterrupted supply can make the difference between life and death. This chapter introduced tools such as the Economic Order Quantity (EOQ) model, ABC analysis, and safety stock calculation as essential methods for controlling inventory. The FEFO (First-Expired, First-Out) principle was explained as particularly vital in healthcare, where medicines and blood products have strict shelf lives. By applying these tools, hospitals can reduce the risks of both shortages and wastage.

This chapter also emphasized the role of digital systems such as the Logistics Management Information System (LMIS), which increase visibility and reduce the human errors common in manual systems. A key lesson here is that while methods such as EOQ and ABC are well established in industry, their application in healthcare must be carefully adapted to account for urgency, patient safety, and the diversity of items stored. Hospitals that adopt these practices can achieve a delicate balance: maintaining the right supplies at the right cost while safeguarding against risks that compromise care.

Chapter 3

Optimizing Hospital Logistics Flows

Flow management encompasses both material and information flows and links. It is crucial in maintaining an efficient patient and material flow, which includes drugs, medical supplies, lab results, test results, medical records, and X-ray results. These resources move through various points as dictated by the established process. Without effective management, inefficiencies can arise in the workflow. The theories applicable to this area include flow diagram design, flow balancing, and flow routing.

Initiating this process requires us to first identify the products circulating within the hospital as shown in Figure 3.1. Let us explore the challenges in managing flow. We focus on three main principles: (1) managing flow diagrams (facility layout), (2) balancing flow (line balancing), and (3) organizing flow paths (routing).

3.1 Flow Diagram Management (Facility Layout)

If a hospital exhibits the following conditions, it may need to address its flow management:

- ➢ areas of congestion, where space is not being fully utilized;
- ➢ excessive stock;
- ➢ extensive distances between processes; or
- ➢ bottlenecks in some processes, while others remain idle.

Food	Patient meals and staff meals
Clothing	General linen, sterile linen, patient attire, operating room staff attire, and staff uniforms
Medications	Inpatient medications per doctor's orders (including take-home medicine, STAT DOSE), ward medications, chemotheray drugs, anesthetics, outpatient medications, and saline, etc.
Medical Supplies	Prescription medical supplies, ward medical supplies, outpatient medical supplies, oxygen tubes, analytical chemicals, and equipment such as surgical gowns, needles, and syringes, etc.
Medical Devices	Various medical devices
Blood and Blood Components	Blood samples and blood components
Specimens	Specimens send to the lab like blood vessels, urine, stool blood samples, Hemoculture, etc.
Parcels	Miscellaneous supplies, forms, office equipment
Patients	Outpatients and inpatients
Waste	General waste, infectious waste, hazardous waste, recyclable waste, and waste requiring autoclave treatment

Figure 3.1. Assortment of products available in hospitals.

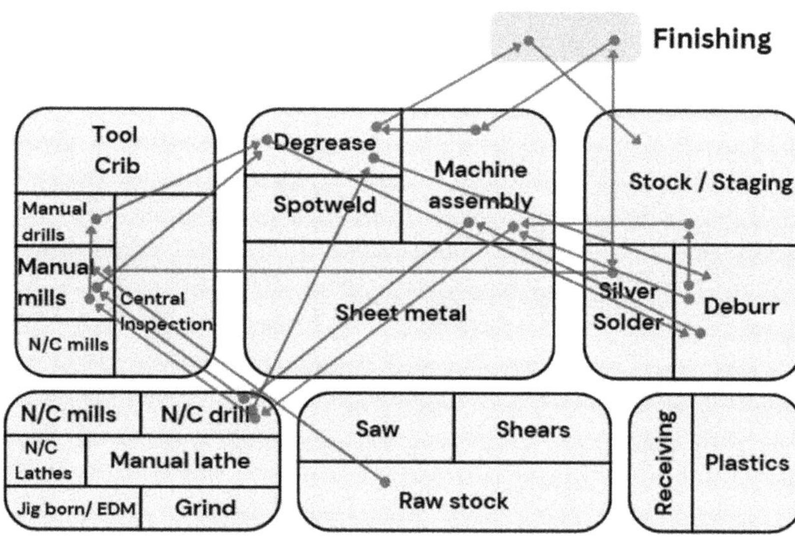

Figure 3.2. Sample flow diagram.

There is a challenge concerning the use of flow diagrams in healthcare settings (see Figure 3.2). Essentially, there are three primary types of flow diagrams frequently observed in hospitals:

(1) Fixed position layout: This layout consists of a stationary workpiece, with personnel, machinery, equipment, and resources gravitating toward it. This approach is typically adopted when space is limited and equipment alterations are made based on the specific nature of the workpiece. Each piece is unique.

(2) Office layout: We use this layout to make the most of the available room space. It starts with identifying the roles of different areas and understanding their interconnections, as shown in Figure 3.3.

Six levels of importance: The chart in this figure illustrates the relationships in an office with five work areas. The president's section, for instance, has the highest level of interaction with the secretary—let's classify this relationship as "A". On the other hand, the president's role exhibits the least interaction with the photocopiers—we can categorize this relationship as "X". This information can be visualized in a diagram, as shown in Figure 3.4, and assist in redesigning the office layout, as depicted in Figure 3.5.

(3) Process-oriented layout: This layout arrangement is frequently used in hospitals. It is a plan that organizes similar processes together to optimize the flow of people and materials. Specifically designed for the new building and hospital logistics.

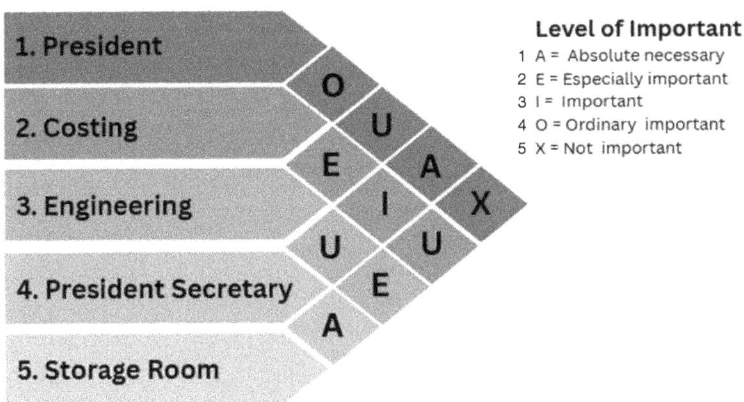

Figure 3.3. Relationship (proximity) chart.

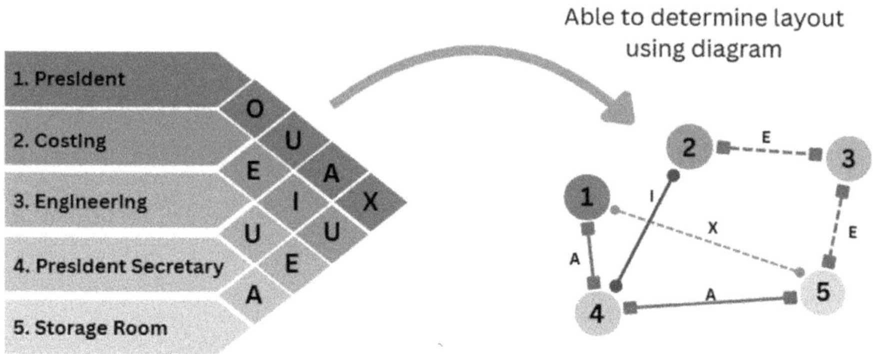

Figure 3.4. Relationship (proximity) chart.

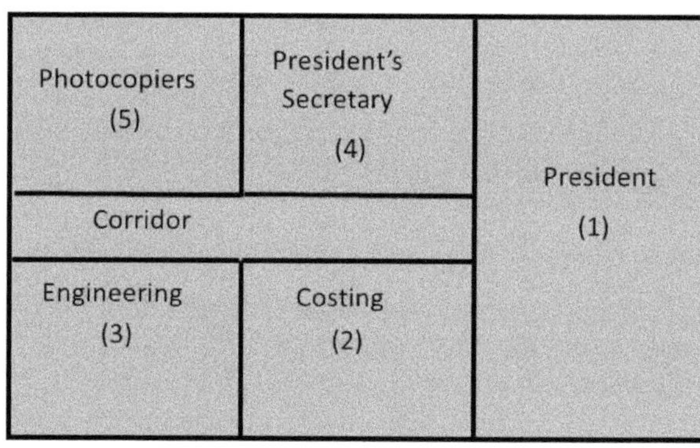

Figure 3.5. Office layout.

String diagram: In this planning approach, our initial step involves gathering data on transport frequencies between agencies. We utilize a from-to chart for this purpose, as shown in Figure 3.6. In the figure, each entry in the table indicates the weekly load shared between departments numbered 1–6. For instance, the frequency of transport from departments 1 to 2 is 40 loads per week, while the return from departments 2 to 1 is 10 loads per week, and so forth. We then sum the frequencies for both outgoing and return journeys between each pair of departments (as shown in Figure 3.6) to achieve the results demonstrated in Figure 3.7.

For better comprehension, the values in Figure 3.8 are represented as a graph in Figure 3.9, as follows.

From \ To	1	2	3	4	5	6
1		40	100	0	0	0
2	10		10	40	10	0
3	0	20		0	0	80
4	0	10	20		50	0
5	0	0	0	0		0
6	20	0	20	0	0	

Figure 3.6. Part flows (loads/week).

Number of loads/week between department	1	2	3	4	5	6
1		50	100	0	0	20
2			30	40	10	0
3				20	0	100
4					50	0
5						0
6						

A = 100
E = 50
I = 10
O = 1
U = 0
X = –100

Figure 3.7. Interdepartmental flow of parts.

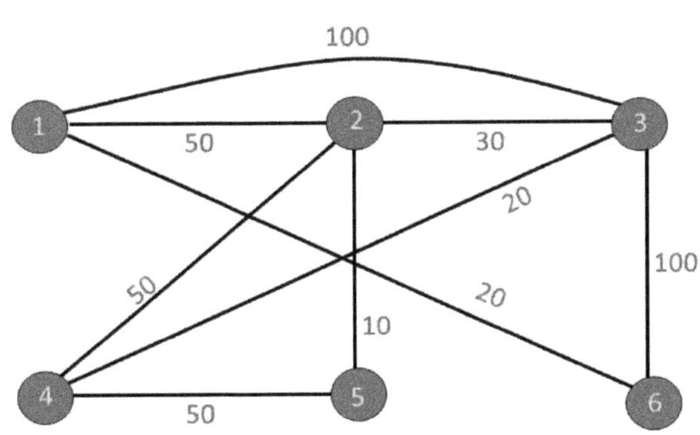

Figure 3.8. Initial layout flow graph indicating loads/week.

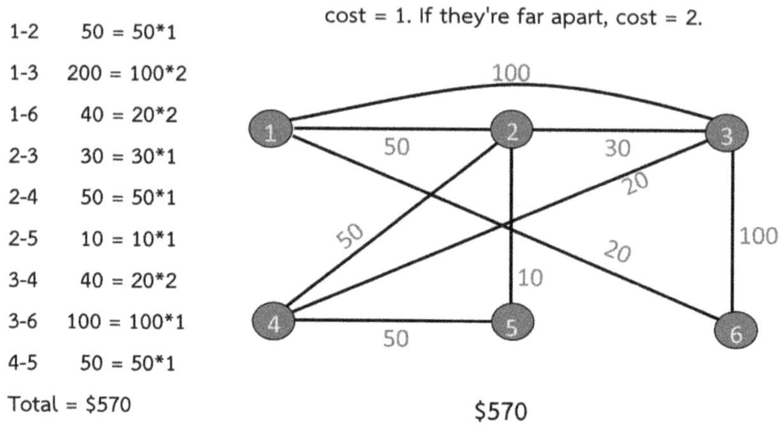

Figure 3.9. Time/cost of initial layout.

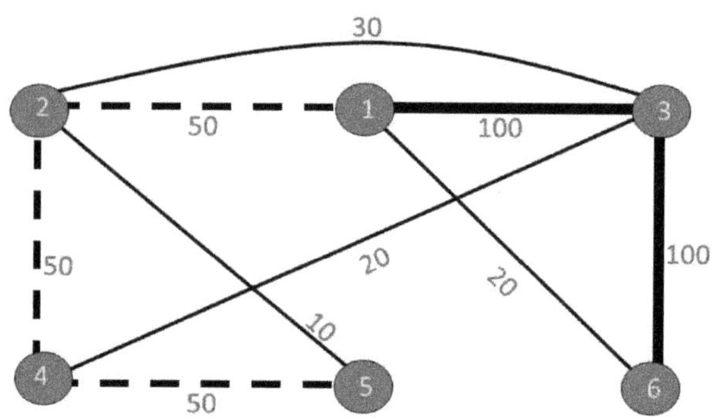

Figure 3.10. Refined layout flow diagram.

To calculate the cost, the value shown in Figure 3.8 is multiplied by a specific weighting factor. We assign cost values based on the distance between transport locations. For nearby locations, a cost of \$1 is assigned, while a cost of \$2 is assigned for those farther apart. The total cost for these settings is \$570, as represented in Figure 3.9.

As depicted in the image, density is observed between units 1–3 and 3–6. We can reorganize the plots for better visibility (as shown in Figure 3.10).

Our findings suggest a potential opportunity to streamline costs by adjusting our existing configurations. As illustrated in the graphic, there is noticeable density between units 1–3 and 3–6. We have

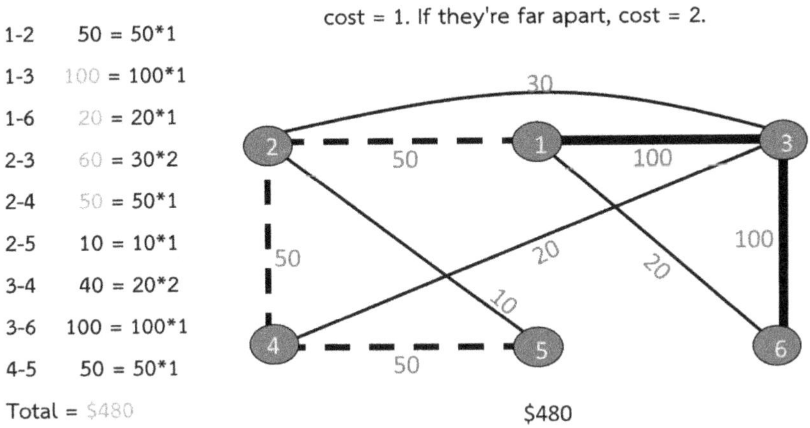

Figure 3.11. Costs from layout improvement.

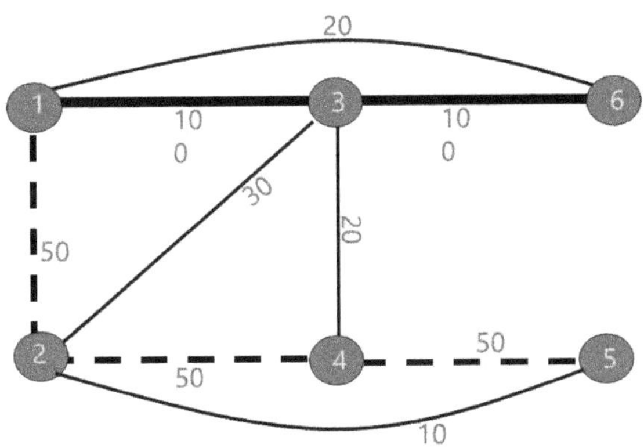

Figure 3.12. An alternative to reduce cross-traffic.

the option to rearrange the plots for improved clarity. Figures 3.11 and 3.12 highlight how a reduced weight factor can yield significant cost efficiencies. This modification offers advantages, enabling us to reduce the cost from its previous level to $480.

A practical method for reducing redundant transport routes would be to eliminate overlaps between routes 2–5, 1–6, and 3–4. Implementing this strategy could potentially reduce costs to $460, as illustrated in Figure 3.12.

3.2 Line Balancing

Flow balancing, or line balancing, involves assigning different subtasks to suitable workstations. The aim is to make the total production time at each station as equal as possible. In this manner, we ensure that no station experiences overburden or underutilization, thereby preventing bottlenecks, work pileups, or excessive wait times. It also reduces idle time at each station. Essentially, this concept of production balancing allows for efficient use of resources such as personnel, machinery, and equipment.

A state of continuous flow is achieved when all stations complete their tasks in an equal amount of time. The objective is to efficiently bundle subtasks (or tasks) at each station to consume a uniform amount of time, such as the 10-minute example provided here (Figure 3.13).

For instance (see Figure 3.14), Station 1 operates task A for 10 minutes. Station 2 operates tasks B and C, each for 5 minutes, for a total of 10 minutes. Similarly, Station 3 operates task D for 2 minutes, E for 3 minutes, and F for 5 minutes, collectively consuming 10 minutes.

3.2.1 *Flow balancing example*

In a single day (8 hours), the goal is to complete 100 pieces of workflow from the process, with each piece involving nine subtasks. from A to I, as shown in Figure 3.15.

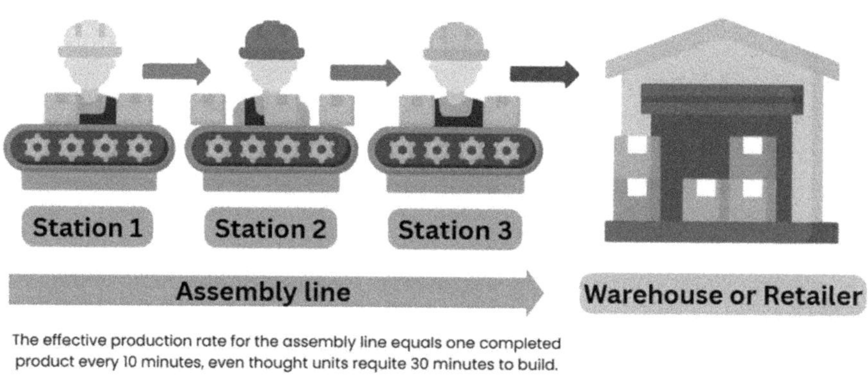

Figure 3.13. Line balancing concept.

A Perfectly-Balance Assembly Line

Station 1 (10 Minutes)	**Station 2** (10 Minutes)	**Station 3** (10 Minutes)	**Total Time** (30 Minutes)
Task A (10 Minutes)	**Task B** (5 Minutes)	**Task D** (2 Minutes)	
	Task C (5 Minutes)	**Task E** (3 Minutes)	**Assume the cycle time is 10 minutes**
		Task F (5 Minutes)	
10 Minutes Productive Time	**10 Minutes** Productive Time	**10 Minutes** Productive Time	**30 Minutes** Total Productive Time
0 Minutes Idle Time	0 Minutes Idle Time	0 Minutes Idle Time	0 Minutes Idle Time

Figure 3.14. The assembly line balancing concept.

Task	Process of previous subtasks.	Standard Time
A	none	60
B	A	80
C	none	30
D	C	40
E	B,D	40
F	none	50
G	F	100
H	D,G	70
I	E,H	30
		Σ = 500 seconds

Figure 3.15. Process of the previous subtasks.

Tasks need to be completed in sequence according to Figure 3.16.

The initial step involves calculating cycle time, defined as the duration a piece of work remains at one station before transitioning to the subsequent station:

$$\text{Cycle time} = \frac{\text{Total time per day}}{\text{Number of pieces required}}.$$

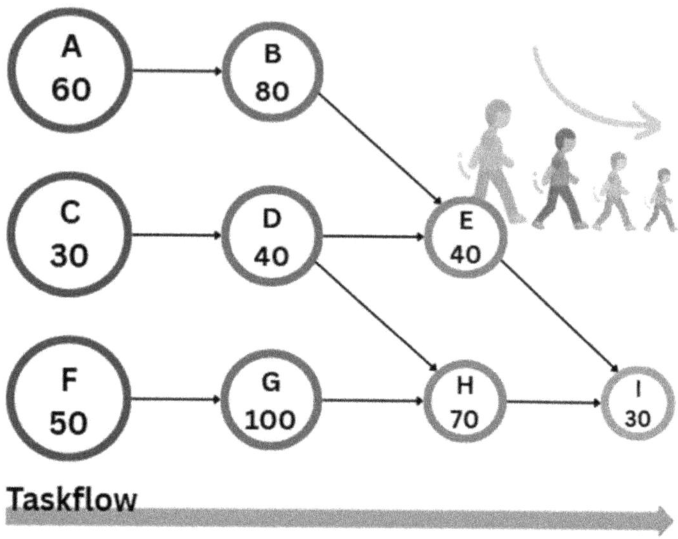

Figure 3.16. Workflow of nine subtasks.

By incorporating relevant values for our example, assuming an eight-hour working day, we could again

$$\begin{aligned}\text{Cycle time} &= \frac{28{,}800\ \text{seconds}}{160\ \text{pieces}}\\ &= 180\ \text{seconds.}\end{aligned}$$

We can establish the number of necessary stations by

$$\begin{aligned}\text{Number of stations} &= \frac{\text{Time required to complete 1 job (9 sub-jobs)}}{\text{Cycle time}}\\ &= \frac{500\ \text{seconds}}{180\ \text{seconds}}\\ &= 2.77 \approx 3\ \text{stations.}\end{aligned}$$

The task at hand is to sort subtasks into three stations, ensuring each station has a cycle time of 180 seconds and prioritizing the steps. (see Figures 3.17 and 3.18.)

Cycle Time	180 Seconds	180 Seconds	180 Seconds	540 Seconds
Production Station	Station 1	Station 2	Station 3	Total
Productive Time Per Cycle				
Idle Time Per Cycle				

Figure 3.17. The line balancing spreadsheet #1.

Cycle Time	180 Seconds	180 Seconds	180 Seconds	540 Seconds
Production Station	Station 1	Station 2	Station 3	Total
Productive Time Per Cycle	**Task A** (60 S)			
Idle Time Per Cycle				

Figure 3.18. The line balancing spreadsheet #2.

Our analysis indicates that balancing the flow in this scenario, with nine subtasks, necessitates three main stations. The cycle time at each station should not exceed 180 seconds. By grouping the subtasks, we can assign as follows (see Figures 3.19 to 3.23):

- Station 1 handles subtasks A, B, and C.
- Station 2 manages subtasks F and G.
- Station 3 takes care of subtasks D, H, E, and I.

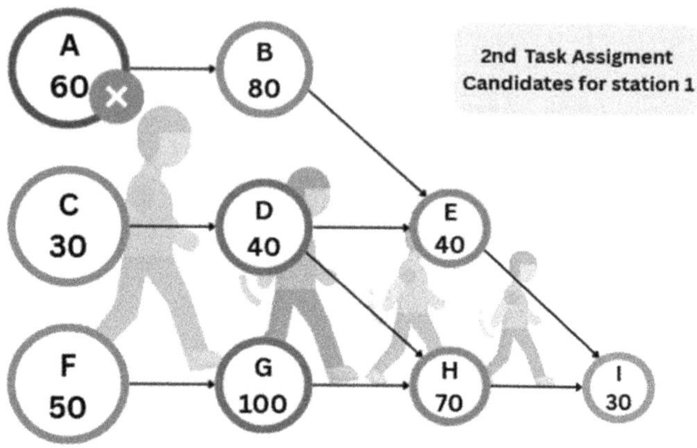

Figure 3.19. The precedence diagram.

Cycle Time	180 Seconds	180 Seconds	180 Seconds	540 Seconds
Production Station	**Station 1**	**Station 2**	**Station 3**	**Total**
Productive Time Per Cycle	**Task A** (60 S) **Task B** (80 S)			
Idle Time Per Cycle				

Figure 3.20. The line balancing spreadsheet #3.

This method allows us to assess work efficiency, which is calculated as

$$\text{Efficiency} = \frac{\text{Total time}}{\text{Actual time used}}$$
$$= \frac{500 \text{ seconds}}{540 \text{ seconds}} = 92.6\%.$$

The complete assignment for Station 1 is detailed in Figures 3.21 and 3.22.

While planning smaller tasks at stations, it is essential to take into account the skill sets of the station staff and potential groupings

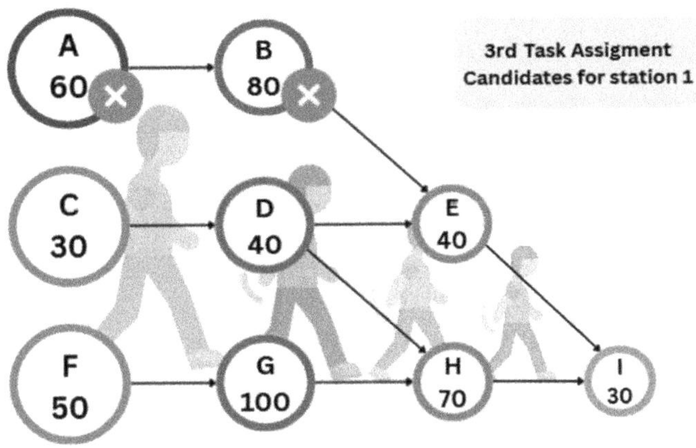

Figure 3.21. The precedence diagram.

Cycle Time	180 Seconds	180 Seconds	180 Seconds	540 Seconds
Production Station	Station 1	Station 2	Station 3	Total
Productive Time Per Cycle	**Task A** (60 S) **Task B** (80 S) **Task C** (30 S)			
Idle Time Per Cycle	**10** Seconds			

Figure 3.22. The line balancing spreadsheet #4.

of tasks. This method proves to be especially useful for service tasks that involve ongoing processes across successive stations. The final line balancing assignment is shown in Figure 3.23.

3.3 Flow Routing

Flow routing is a tool for managing logistics within healthcare settings. Its primary function is to identify the most efficient routes when there are numerous orders to fulfill. In this context, efficiency

Cycle Time	180 Seconds	180 Seconds	180 Seconds	540 Seconds
Production Station	**Station 1**	**Station 2**	**Station 3**	**Total**
Productive Time Per Cycle	**Task A** (60 S) **Task B** (60 S) **Task C** (60 S)	**Task F** (50 S) **Task G** (100 S)	**Task D** (40 S) **Task H** (70 S) **Task E** (40 S) **Task I** (30 S)	**500** Seconds
Idle Time Per Cycle	**10** Seconds	**30** Seconds	**0** Seconds	**40** Seconds

Figure 3.23. The line balancing spreadsheet #5.

is a measure of cost and distance. Applications of flow routing can vary from delivering orders from the dispensing unit to the recipient, receiving orders back to the dispensing unit, or facilitating interdepartmental deliveries.

3.3.1 *There are two main scenarios for the delivery and receipt of goods*

(1) Pure pickup/pure delivery (Figure 3.24) refers to the separate rounds of delivering and receiving products.
(2) Mixed pickup/mixed delivery (Figure 3.25) means that products are delivered and received simultaneously. This scenario can be further categorized into three cases:

   (a) Separate routes, with one round for delivery and another for receiving.
   (b) One route, not interspersed, where the delivery and pickup occur in the same cycle but are not intermingled.
   (c) Interspersed delivery refers to a system in which the delivery and receipt of goods occur simultaneously.

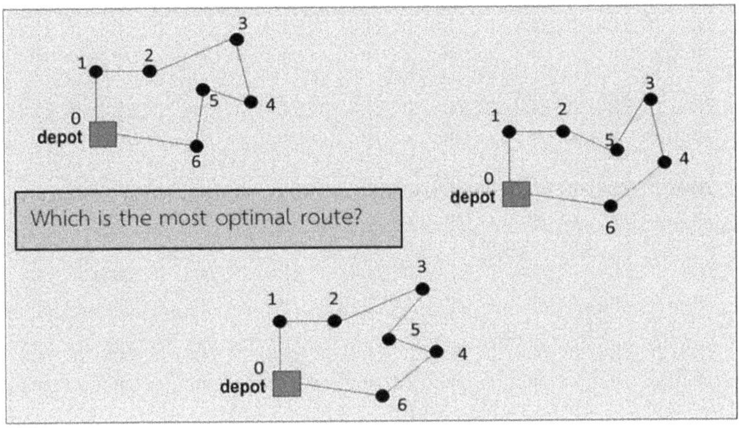

Figure 3.24. Pure pickup or delivery.

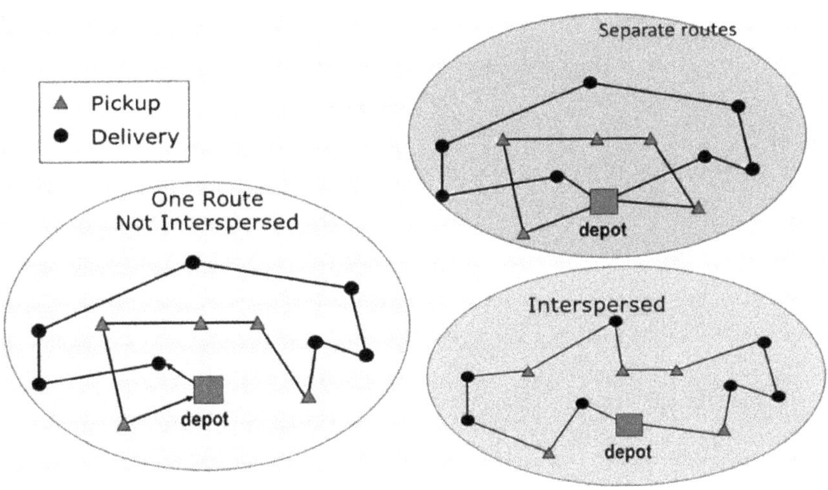

Figure 3.25. Mixed pickup and delivery.

There are two types of principles used in route design (Figure 3.26):

(1) The Travelling Salesman Problem (TSP), or Milk Run, involves delivering to every point in a single transport cycle.
(2) The Vehicle Routing Problem (VRP) involves dividing transport zones and then arranging routes.

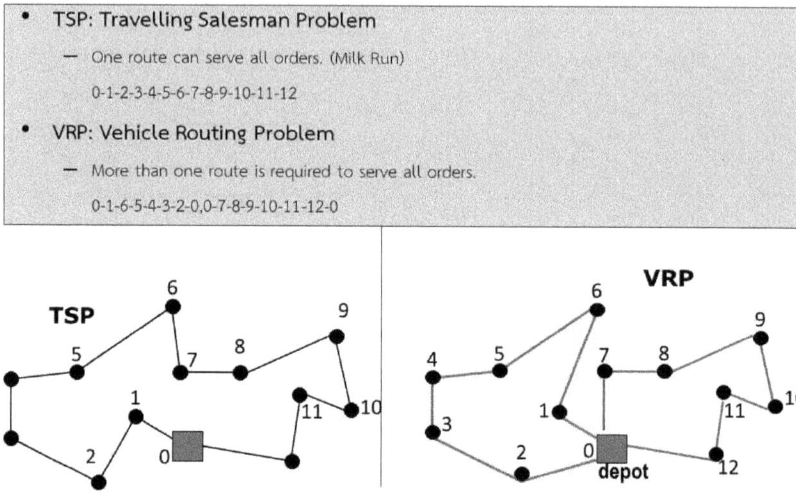

Figure 3.26. TSP and VRP.

In designing transportation routes, we use two simple transport sequencing formats: the Nearest Neighbor Heuristic and the Nearest Insertion Heuristic:

1. **Nearest Neighbor heuristic:** This approach involves determining the travel path of transport vehicles by selecting the shortest route from a company (DC) to various customers. The default route begins with the company and proceeds to the nearest customer. Then, the closest unassigned customer on the list is selected, and this process continues until all customers are assigned to a route without exceeding the vehicle's capacity. If the total demand exceeds the vehicle's capacity, the current route is closed, and the process restarts until all customers are covered.
2. **Nearest Insertion heuristic:** This approach is suitable for routing with a large amount of transport data and varying delivery deadlines. However, given the limited number of vehicles available, priority must be given to the most urgent transportation tasks. Before the deadline, the latest delivery date (or latest due date) and remaining time (or slack time) are considered. After that, the necessary work is organized into transportation routes by insertion into each vehicle, considering the total distance value, the

vehicle capacity, and the delivery timeframe. The process repeats until all transport tasks are placed on the route.

3.4 The Supply, Processing, and Distribution (SPD) Concept in Hospital Logistics

A new dimension of hospital transportation management is introduced with the Supply, Processing, and Distribution (SPD) concept, improving the efficiency of inventory management and transportation systems within the hospital.

Challenges of hospital logistics are as follows:

1. Many have identified management issues as a major hurdle within hospitals. These include problems with inventory, transportation systems, and information technology systems.
2. There is an overstock of inventory with an average shelf life of 1.5–2 months. This results in items expiring before they can be used and a lack of storage space. Occasionally, there are shortages, leading to insufficient supplies. These issues stem from a lack of data synchronization between the warehouse and the service unit. The warehouse is unaware of the service unit's usage and inventory levels. Moreover, the transportation system is inefficient, with units collecting their goods from the warehouse at set times.

3.4.1 *What is the Supply, Processing, and Distribution (SPD) agency?*

The SPD agency is essentially a central agency that functions much like a logistics service provider, also known as third-party logistics (3PLs) provider. Its main responsibility is the management of a hospital's inventory and warehouse, including the transportation and distribution of products to various units within the hospital.

In addition to these duties, the SPD also serves as an information hub, ensuring smooth product flow, optimal control, and minimal logistics costs. This includes managing essential data, such as product usage forecasts and reserve plans for different departments, and ensuring that supply meets demand under both normal and emergency conditions. Furthermore, this agency can plan product transportation and distribution for maximum efficiency.

The SPD agency can be either established within the hospital or outsourced.

3.4.1.1 *Supply Processing and Distribution (SPD)*

With the evolving role of logistics activities, the establishment of an SPD agency will inevitably impact information exchange among existing members. For instance, establishing an SPD agency would enable it to act on behalf of the Treasury, establish links, and exchange information with other members.

The details of how the establishment of an SPD agency would affect information exchange among members of the public health supply chain are as follows (Figure 3.27).

(1) Relationship between the SPD agency and hospitals

The SPD agency will partner with the hospital in two main activities:

(a) *Activity: Initiate withdrawal requests via the requisition note or product transfer request form.* Originally, agencies sent these requests to the warehouse via a bill of lading or product transfer request form. However, this is changing as SPD agencies are now

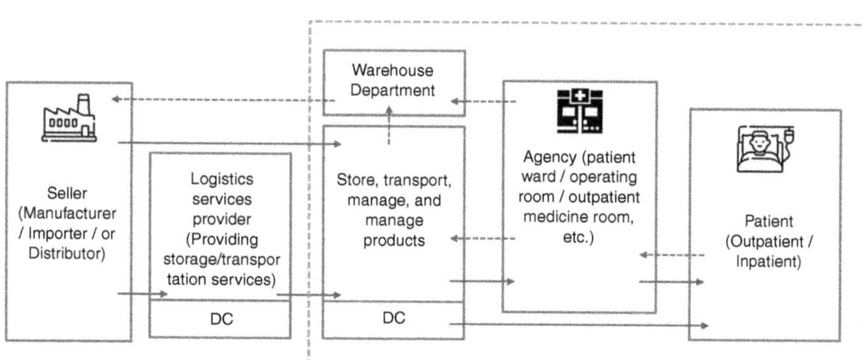

Figure 3.27. Linking and exchanging information between members of the public health supply chain if an SPD agency is established.

required to verify the actual consumption or remaining balance across various agencies using one of three methods:

- Establish a data connection (interface) between the agency's IT system and the SPD's IT system.
- The SPD deploys its representatives to evaluate actual departmental expenditures.
- The agency personnel assess their own agency's actual usage or remaining balance and communicate this information to the SPD agency.

(b) *Activity: Product transport.* Conventionally, product transportation fell into two categories: either the agency collected the product from the warehouse or the warehouse delivered the products to the agency. Now, with the advent of the SPD agency, it will handle transportation responsibilities.

(2) Coordination between the SPD department and the hospital's warehouse department

The SPD will manage inventory, estimate product demand, and relay this information to the supplies department. This communication will streamline purchasing and sales contract processes, including the issuance of product purchase orders.

(3) Interaction between the hospital's warehouse department and the seller

The warehouse department will issue product sales contracts for necessary items based on the forecast data on product usage that the SPD sends to the hospital's warehouse department.

The warehouse department will use this data to gauge the quantity of product usage during each period, such as weekly or monthly, and issue product purchase orders accordingly. When the product is delivered to the SPD agency, the seller should include the delivery note/tax invoice. The SPD agency will then document the product receipt in the IT system. The advance provision of product delivery details by the seller will assist the SPD agency in planning product receipts more efficiently.

(4) Relationship between the distributor (or distribution center, DC) and SPD

The connection between DC and SPD is a recent development. It is supervised by a logistics service provider who manages the products' logistics processes from upstream to downstream. Upstream, the distributor (DC) collects products from various sellers; downstream, SPD acts as a hub-and-spoke unit, distributing products to users at various payment points. The actual usage data or remaining balance at the payment points are required as initial data to manage the number of products at SPD and meet the needs of the dispensing points.

3.4.2 *Guidelines to incorporate information and adapt operational procedures post SPD agency establishment*

Operational procedures revised after the initiation of an SPD agency

The product disbursement process involves the SPD agency gathering product usage data. It includes calculating the top-up amount, arranging products, transporting products, reporting replenishment results, and storing products. All these processes benefit from the E-Kanban concept (Figure 3.28), which aids in planning and product replenishment across various departments in the hospital.

When a product is used, the associated *Kanban* is compiled by the agency and stored in a designated place. SPD units then journey to each department to collect used *Kanban*, facilitating data collection and replenishment calculations. Replenishment equals the quantity of *Kanban* used. The frequency of product replenishment may need to be discussed. *Kanban* data are electronically transmitted and linked with the established information program system. When the SPD agency restocks the products at the agency (Figure 3.29), a new *Kanban* is attached to each product and stored in its original place.

The product ordering process involves the SPD agency checking the SPD warehouse product balance and calculating product purchase requests. This process considers total product usage, withdrawal departments, trends, and product stock reserves (buffer or safety stock). The traditional method of submitting product order

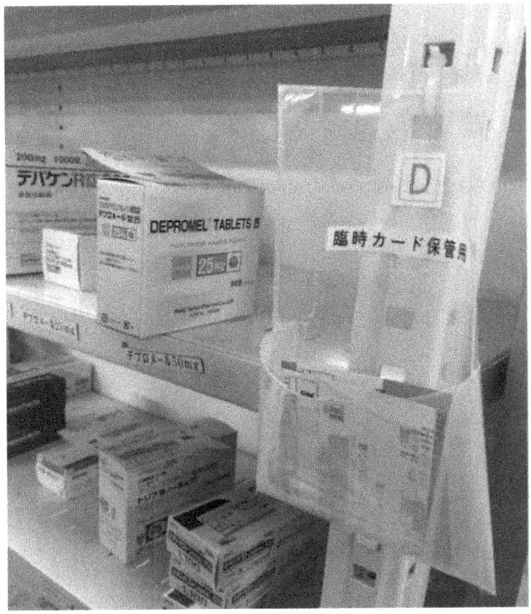

Figure 3.28. Illustration of *Kanban* attached to a product and used for product replenishment.

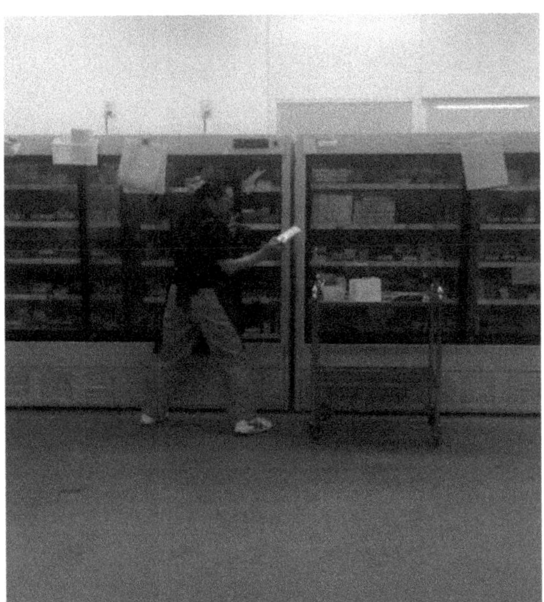

Figure 3.29. SPD agency restocking products at the department.

documents is replaced with electronic submission through the Electronic Data Interchange (EDI) system. Sellers can confirm product delivery in the SPD's information system, connected to the EDI system, by specifying the product delivery date to the SPD warehouse and confirming readiness for product inspection.

The product tracking and replenishment process involves coordination between the DC and SPD warehouses. This vendor-managed inventory process has the DC monitor each SPD warehouse's product usage and plan product replenishment, while also notifying the hospital to issue a purchase order for that product.

The SPD unit is tasked with reporting daily product usage to the DC distributor, who then monitors the product usage status, calculates replenishment quantities, arranges products, and continues product deliveries to the SPD.

3.4.3 *List of potential benefits*

(1) For manufacturer/distributor

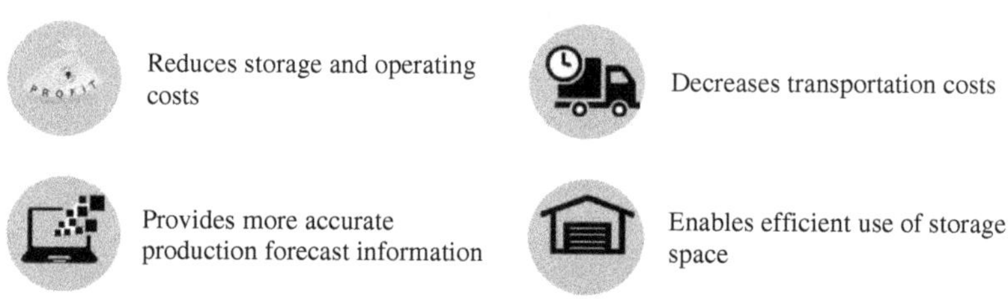

Note: It also lowers the cost of hiring employees and minimizes wasted time due to inexperience.

(2) For hospital

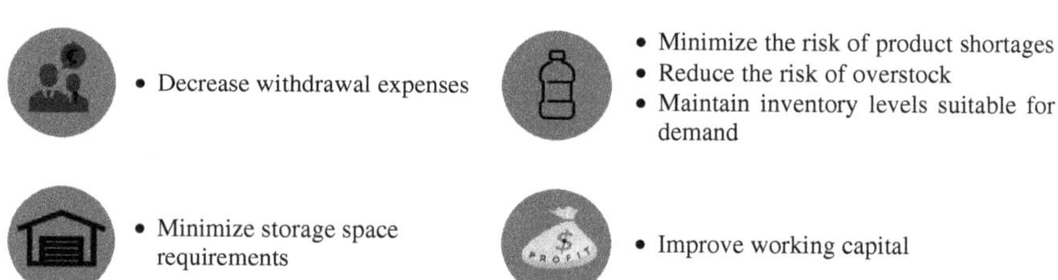

Note: Allocate resources efficiently based on expertise.

3.5 Centralized Inter-Hospital Warehousing and Smart Platform Integration[1]

Innovative Concept[1]: The establishment of a central warehouse between hospitals and the development of an in-warehouse platform system. This would employ modern technology to aid logistics systems, medications, and medical supplies.

The healthcare industry in Thailand is predicted to grow from $76.63 million in 2022 to $600.89 million by 2030. With more than 1,000 public hospitals, Thailand's expansive healthcare industry is complemented by 300 private hospitals offering a broad scope of treatment with modern facilities. Currently, enhancing quality and patient safety is a significant focus in the medical field. Despite continued development in Thailand's public health services, gaps in the health service system persist, largely due to supply chain complications. Most hospitals struggle with inventory management and logistics, primarily because their information technology systems function separately. These issues can result in excessive inventory buildup, with most hospitals storing supplies for an average of 1.5–2 months. This frequently causes some medicines or medical products to expire before they can be used. Additionally, certain products may not have enough storage space, leading to occasional shortages that affect usage. The current system for transporting products within the hospital relies on self-transportation, where staff from each unit must collect products from various warehouses throughout the hospital.

Looking at the storage facilities within hospitals, they tend to be fragmented, with separate warehouses for drugs, medical supplies, fabrics, and sterile medical supplies (Figure 3.30). These decentralized warehouses each have their own inventory management, warehouse management, and transportation systems. This is consistent across all hospitals, including those within a network, which still operate separate warehouses. On the selling company's side, if a company has more than one group of products (including drugs/medical supplies) that need to be delivered to hospitals, those products must be delivered to various warehouses within separate hospital buildings.

[1]This section is modified from Kanjanapachara *et al.* (2024), a centralized distribution center offers solutions to common inventory challenges in hospitals, pp. 1034–1036.

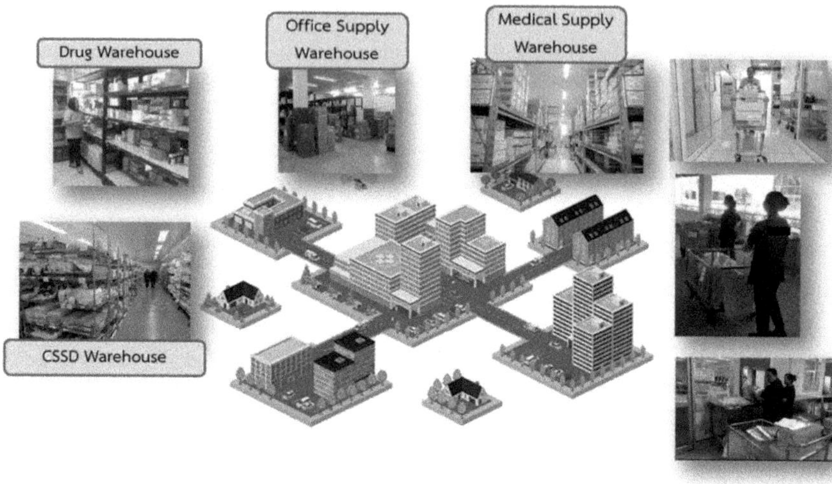

Figure 3.30. Decentralized warehouse in a hospital.

This requires the hospital to allocate personnel resources to manage separate warehouses for different product groups, which can significantly impact hospital costs. On a district, provincial, or regional level, managing separate warehouses in every hospital results in a considerable amount of stock.

Our preliminary study on the cost–benefit of a central warehouse project for hospitals has resulted in the design of drug and medical supply management activities. This includes the introduction of a distribution center to store and distribute products to service points. We have proposed three new models, with details as follows (see Figure 3.31 for diagrams of these models):

Current Model (AS-IS): This model starts when various manufacturers deliver products to the hospital's drug and medical supply warehouse. The hospital's warehouse then distributes these products to different points of use. At these points, staff members will collect these products from the warehouse.

Proposed Model 1 (TO-BE1): In this model, the distribution center manages inventory instead of the drug and medical supply warehouse. The hospital's warehouse only serves as a stopping point, responsible for receiving products from the distribution center and distributing them to the points of use.

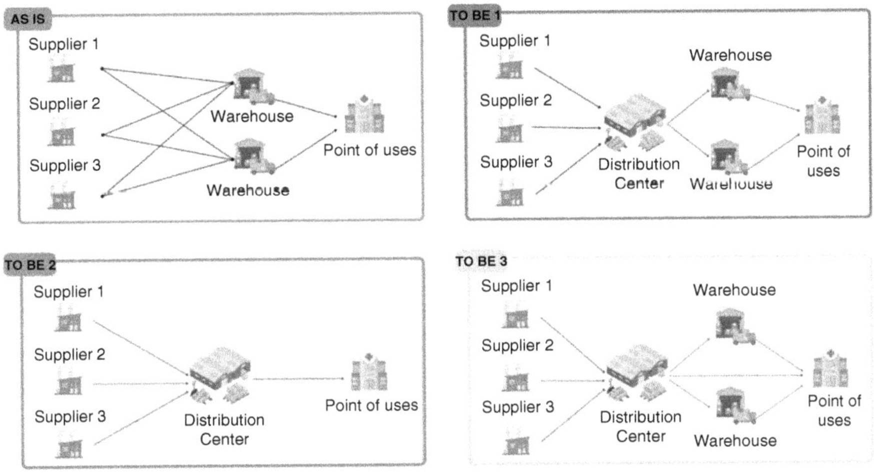

Figure 3.31. Redesigning the flow of drug and medical supply management with the integration of a distribution center (DC).

Source: Modified from Kanjanapachara *et al.* (2024), a centralized distribution center offers solutions to common inventory challenges in hospitals (pp. 1034–1036).

Proposed Model 2 (TO-BE2): This model eliminates the need for a hospital drug or medical supply warehouse. Instead, a distribution center manages inventory and transports it directly to points of use.

Proposed Model 3 (TO-BE3): This model proposes transporting medicines and medical supplies from distribution centers based on usage frequency. High-demand items are transported directly from the distribution center to the point of use. For low- or no-demand items, the distribution center transports goods to holding points, which then distribute the product to points of use.

The key performance indicators used in our calculations included logistics costs (comprising operating costs, transportation costs, and holding costs), the value of goods stuck in the hospital warehouse, warehouse operation time, and waiting times. The results showed that the new Proposed Model 3 is the most suitable for the hospital context. Compared to other models, this model allows for simpler modifications to the working model. It reduces logistics costs by 18% compared to the current model and improves the waiting time for goods from an unstable 0–15 days to a consistent 1 day.

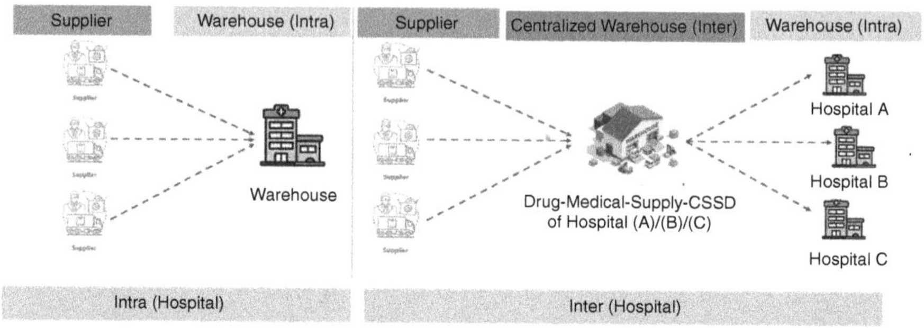

Figure 3.32. Comparison between traditional transportation and centralized warehousing transportation.

Consequently, we are considering the development of a centralized warehouse connecting different hospitals, with the assistance of modern technology. The idea is to establish a central distribution center for products used across the network or within hospitals in the same area (Figure 3.32 illustrates this comparison). This offsite warehouse will free up valuable hospital space for other uses, such as adding beds or examination rooms. It will also help cut costs related to management, inventory, and storage, thereby enhancing the efficiency of inventory management, warehousing, and transportation systems. This will lead to improved service quality in the public health system and the country's health industry, better quality of life for the public, continuous access to quality medicines, reduced travel issues related to postal medication delivery, more job opportunities in warehouse or distribution center areas, and decreased carbon dioxide emissions resulting from efficient transportation.

We plan to utilize technology and digital innovation to create a platform for managing central warehouses between hospitals and intelligent hospital drug transport systems. The focus will be on nearby hospitals or those within the same network. The platform under development will cover critical warehouse activities such as order receipt, pick preparation, packing, and transport preparation. The system will support and integrate with various modern technologies, such as the Automated Storage/Retrieval System (AS/RS), Automated Guided Vehicle (AGV), automatic palletizing, and automatic picking and sorting. Our system will facilitate connections to the smart hospital drug transport system, serving as a central warehouse between hospitals. This platform will manage the distribution of hospital networks in Bangkok and surrounding areas. Not only can it interface with various hospital systems, but it is also compatible with modern technologies such as the AS/RS, AGV, and the Transportation Management System (TMS). If the prototype model of using a central warehouse between hospitals proves successful, there is potential to further develop this system, expanding its reach to provincial and regional levels.

3.6 Conclusion

Efficient logistics flows are the lifeblood of a hospital. This chapter explored how the design of hospital layouts, the movement of goods and patients, and support systems such as porters determine operational effectiveness. Using flow diagrams, managers can visualize processes and identify bottlenecks that cause unnecessary delays. Case studies showed that even small adjustments to specimen transport routes or facility layouts can significantly improve the speed and safety of operations.

The key lesson from this chapter is that hospital logistics flows must be treated as dynamic systems that evolve with changes in demand, staffing, or infrastructure. Continuous monitoring and adjustments ensure that processes remain efficient. Moreover, hospitals must balance the need for speed with the requirement for safety. The examples demonstrated that carefully planned workflows not only save time and resources but also improve the quality of patient care by minimizing risks during the transport of critical supplies.

Chapter 4

Action Plan for Enhancing Hospital Logistics

4.1 Resource (Material/Resource) Management Action Plan

The resource (material/resource) management action plan involves ensuring that resources such as medicines and medical supplies are available in sufficient quantities. Effective management starts at the grassroots level with small medicine rooms, wards, and departments documenting their usage. Precise records of consumption and receipt are crucial. These data are then shared with the main warehouse to facilitate timely replenishment. This leads to an auto-replenishment system, making inventory management a more straightforward process. This type of management simplifies the process. When users are connected through an information system, all they need to do is record their usage. The system updates with each day's balance, allowing those who replenish the stock to see the remaining balance and provide the needed items. This approach makes inventory management more effective and accurate, matching the usage rate without the need for excessive stock. It also reduces the risk of running out of stock. To implement this, users should track the movement of materials—such as drugs and medical supplies—recording how much was withdrawn and used. This can be entered into the system at the end of the cycle or day, replacing the need for a disbursement book. The main warehouse or the person replenishing the products can then see the balance and restock accordingly.

In addition, the person replenishing the stock (e.g., in the medicine room) should record the used amount and the amount for replenishment. This ensures accurate and efficient inventory management. With this method, inventory at various points, such as medicine warehouses, patient wards, delivery rooms, and emergency rooms, rotates faster. It prevents overstocking and addresses the problem of expired products.

Utilizing technology, such as barcodes, to scan receipts and payments from the system can enhance accuracy. This reduces the recording process and increases patient safety. For example, when recording patient information and dispensing medicines, scanning barcodes can ensure the correct medication is administered to the right patient in a timely manner. This practice can significantly improve patient safety.

Implementing automatic inventory management (Auto-replenishment) from point of use to supplier—for instance, from ward/Out Patient Department (OPD) to medicine room, from medicine room to warehouse, and from warehouse to supplier—can streamline supply chain management through Vendor-Managed Inventory (VMI). This system enables efficient replenishment of stock from the medicine room to the ward, from the medicine warehouse to the medicine room, from the medicine warehouse to the Subdistrict Health Promoting Hospital in the network, and from suppliers to drug warehouses.

Restocking medicine warehouses at the subdistrict health promoting hospital can be done in the same way (Figure 4.1). The hospital records the amount used and sends it to the primary hospital. The primary hospital can then decide to replenish the stock, ensuring there are no shortages or excesses. By managing the delivery of items more efficiently and reducing steps, the primary hospital can send the purchase amount to the supplier, specifying a set of purchase items for each Subdistrict Health Promoting Hospital. The supplier can then deliver the set to each Subdistrict Health Promoting Hospital. This system, known as cross-docking, means that delivered medicines and medical supplies do not need to be packaged at the main warehouse. Each delivery can then be forwarded without having to be stored in the main warehouse. If storage is necessary, it should be for as little time as possible.

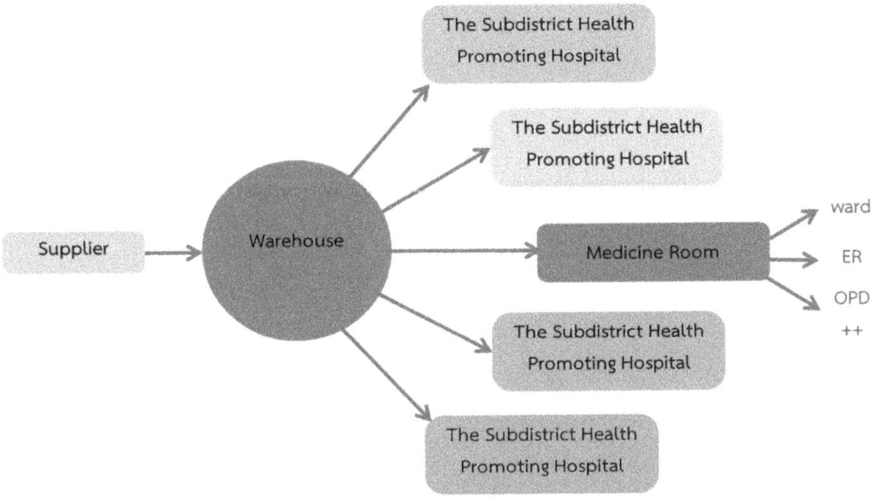

Figure 4.1. Drug flow from the supplier to the point of use.
Source: Adapted from Hospital logistics management (p. 55), by D. Kritchanchai and S. Srisakunwan, 2023, Healthcare Supply Chain Excellence Centre (LogHealth), Mahidol University.

4.2 Reverse Logistics Management of Drugs and Medical Supplies

In terms of reverse logistics, hospitals return medicines from various service units, such as wards and emergency rooms, to the original warehouse. This could be from the ward to the OPD medicine room, Inpatient Department (IPD) medicine room, or from the OPD and IPD medicine rooms back to the medicine warehouse, etc. This return of medicines and medical supplies is influenced by changes in inventory levels, i.e., inventory figures in the information system do not match those in actual storage. This affects inventory planning and can cause the hospital's purchasing plans or estimates of actual usage to be incorrect. Therefore, to ensure the information is accurate and current, the percentage stock accuracy of drugs and medical supplies must be increased. Workers must also record returns, which should be treated the same as normal disbursements, to make inventory levels as accurate as possible. The hospital's purchasing planning section must calculate inventory balances to cover drugs and medical supplies stored in various departments in order to maintain a complete balance. However, there must also be a forecast of the rate of use of drugs and medical supplies within the hospital to reduce the risk of product shortages due to the relatively long purchasing cycle time. In addition to this, hospitals should have indicators for percentage stock accuracy of balances and estimates compared with actual usage numbers in order to continually improve and develop the accuracy of purchasing planning.

4.3 The Sub-Action Plans Suitable for Resource Management

4.3.1 *Material Inventory Management and Purchasing Action Plan*

This involves an electronic data exchange system that covers the sending of purchase orders and delivery notes between hospitals and suppliers. The aim is to increase efficiency and reduce costs in managing inventory and purchasing for maximum benefit. The steps involved for hospitals and suppliers are as follows:

(1) Study the current product ordering and delivery process to identify and rectify any obstacles. This process should be modified to support the exchange of electronic data.
(2) Develop and modify information technology systems that support electronic product ordering and delivery.
(3) Select suitable products for electronic ordering and delivery. These products should have a consistent usage rate and a reasonable price.
(4) Define product code mapping to link electronic data between various departments, warehouses, and suppliers.
(5) Analyze the usage rate of each product type from past usage data to determine the appropriate and sufficient level of products necessary for service provision.
(6) Determine methods for replenishing products each time, such as Min-Max or Material Requirements Planning (MRP), to reduce the risk of product shortages.

(7) Set indicators for electronic product ordering and delivery, such as reduction in product shortages, decreased inventory levels, and faster ordering and delivery cycles.
(8) Train relevant personnel to understand the new processes developed and implement this action plan.
(9) Measure and evaluate performance and improve the ordering and delivery process to enhance efficiency.

The Inventory Management and Purchasing Action Plan is designed to reduce inventory levels and accelerate the ordering and delivery process. However, if hospitals are not yet ready to exchange information electronically, preliminary work can be done by sending information via email. As product code mapping evolves, the transition to electronic data exchange can be made gradually.

4.3.2 *Transportation Management Action Plan*

This plan aims to enhance the efficiency of goods transportation within the hospital by applying the "milk run" technique. In this strategy, transportation units collect goods from various workstations and deliver them during a single trip. For instance, they might pick up clean clothes from the laundry and distribute them to different wards, the outpatient medicine room, and the delivery room. This approach aims to resolve the issue of different departments individually collecting products from the same origin. The steps involved are as follows:

(1) Assess the workload in goods transportation, including the frequency, covered goods, origin, destination, distance, and resources used, such as personnel and transportation carts.
(2) Analyze the product usage rates in each department to determine the appropriate product list and stock levels to prevent product shortages.
(3) Analyze the frequency to determine the suitable number of transport trips each day based on the workload.
(4) Examine the transportation route for each trip to decide the order of delivery to various stations, such as the laundry, ward, emergency room, and delivery room.
(5) Evaluate the number of personnel required for goods transportation, which might involve hiring new staff.

(6) Design or modify transport vehicle packaging boxes to suit the transportation needs, such as using plastic boxes with straps an electric vehicle.
(7) Implement information technology to monitor product usage and to provide more accurate and timely information. This also helps in analyzing the quantity of products that need to be replenished during each trip.

The "milk run" technique focuses on maximizing the value of each transportation trip. Each day, various departments prepare and place the required products at a designated point, and the delivery truck collects them, eliminating the need for empty return trips. This improves the use of transportation vehicles. Initially, there may not be a designated person for transportation. Hospitals can organize shifts, for example, the ward might be responsible on Monday and the emergency room on Tuesday.

4.3.3 *Setting Up a Logistics Agency Action Plan*

A logistics agency, serving as a central unit for the hospital, is responsible for goods movement, collection, procurement, packaging, storage, and distribution. The objective is to ensure products are received and delivered with maximum efficiency and effectiveness. Here are the steps for setting up a hospital logistics unit:

(1) Study the scope of work for the logistics agency that suits the hospital context. This involves determining the framework for the range of product items that the logistics agency should handle.
(2) Allocate personnel based on the workload framework of the logistics agency.
(3) Analyze guidelines for developing the logistics unit within the hospital, potentially partnering with an external logistics company.
(4) Implement information technology for planning and forecasting product demand, replenishing products, tracking products, and managing inventory.
(5) Develop knowledge for logistics agency personnel to enhance efficiency in their roles.

(6) Develop suitable indicators for warehouse management, inventory, and product delivery, such as inventory levels, incidence of product shortages, and faster product delivery times.

Establishing a logistics unit helps reduce costs and duplication and increases efficiency in logistics processes. The logistics systems mentioned are easy to operate, accurate, safe, and efficient. If all systems use the same information language throughout the supply chain (standard data), barcode data must be used from the supplier to the warehouse, drug room, ward, and patient. By linking all data to the same common language, a traceability system (Traceability) can be created. This allows users to check which medicine or medical supplies used for a particular patient came from which batch, which box in the medicine room, which lot from the medicine warehouse, and from which supplier. Expiry date information will also be displayed. If there are any issues with drugs or medical supplies, they can be recalled and traced back to the exact source, maximizing patient safety.

The logistics system can be divided into phases as shown in Figure 4.2.

Logistics activities suitable for application in hospitals can be summarized into five activities (Figure 4.3):

1. **Demand forecasting** involves predicting the demand for drugs and medical supplies. It relies on mathematical models that calculate historical usage data and qualitative methods to improve the accuracy of usage rates. As the ordering process for hospitals takes time, accurate usage forecasts reduce the risk of urgent orders, borrowing medicines, and overstocking.
2. **Order processing** is currently handled by most departments through writing product picking slips and delivering them to the warehouse. To enhance efficiency, hospitals should consider utilizing computer systems and electronic management, such as online withdrawals, balance checks, and product ordering.
3. **Inventory management** is crucial, as it significantly impacts hospital funding. Although having a variety of products can cater well to the needs of service users, it can also consume considerable storage space and tie up capital. Therefore, effective inventory management can help ensure adequate product availability, meet

(1) Short-term: 6 months

- Data sharing management using existing information technology
- Recording usage and receipt in the system and online to stock replenishers
- Starting the Auto Replenishment system by the automatic replenisher
- Studying the work process and eliminating/reducing redundant and unnecessary steps

(2) Medium-term: 1 year

- Introducing technology to assist the above system, such as Barcode
- Linking the Auto Replenishment system to Suppliers (Vendor Managed Inventory - VMI) and Subdistrict Health Promoting Hospitals (Sor. Por. Por.) in the network

(3) Long-term: 3 years

- Creating a logistics and supply chain system in the community hospital network to link data that is the same standard to each other (Standard Data and Supply Chain Network)

Figure 4.2. The action plan for implementing a logistics system in phases.

the needs of service users, minimize the risk of temporary product shortages, and prevent product deterioration or expiration.

4. **Warehouse and storage management** is important due to limited space in hospitals. Most hospitals lack sufficient warehouse space for storing medicines and medical supplies, leading to inefficiency. This inefficiency prolongs the picking and disbursement process. Therefore, effective warehouse management strategies, such as using appropriate racks for storage, labeling storage locations, separating zones for different items, and controlling production batches, are crucial. These strategies help reduce space

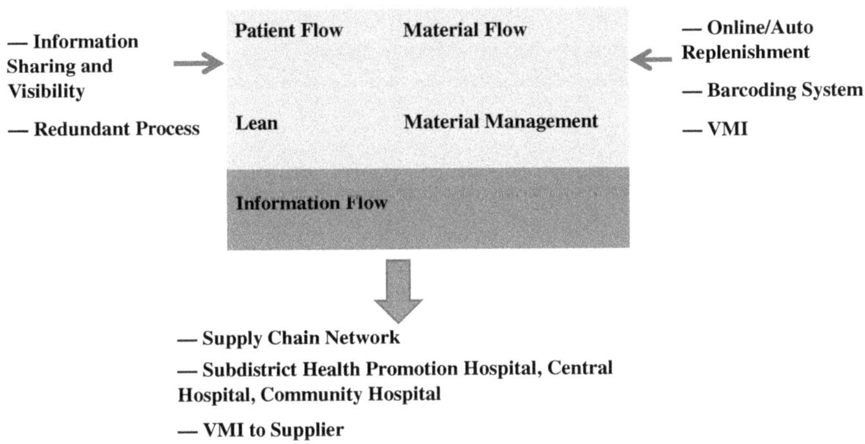

Figure 4.3. Diagram of the logistics system implementation process.

usage, lower the rate of expired products, and speed up the picking process. Additionally, the application of information systems in warehouse management is also important.

5. **Transportation management** is crucial in hospitals due to the variety of products used, including medicines, medical supplies, clothing, and patient food. These items often rely on either the originating or destination agency for transportation, which can lead to inefficiencies. To improve this, transportation could be planned in the form of trips or rounds. The milk run transportation technique could also be utilized to enhance efficiency, reduce workload, and decrease the number of trips per day. It can mitigate the risk of some departments not receiving enough products while others have an excess. However, it is important to adjust transportation equipment, such as carts, delivery vehicles, and containers, to suit the transportation of various types of goods.

When implementing logistics systems, it is important to understand that logistics and supply chain management are not solutions to individual departmental problems. Instead, they are a logistics "**process**" for problem-solving, involving every department and functioning in a connected manner. Therefore, the application of logistics should begin at the establishment level with a cross-functional team, including representatives from each department.

The team should focus on solving prioritized process problems, considering the entire loop, or the End-to-End process. This process involves understanding where it begins, where it ends, and who is involved. Additionally, the team should review and re-engineer the process as a whole system. Clear committees and responsible personnel should be established at the onset of the project. Success indicators and goals should be set, and the project's progress should be regularly evaluated.

Once strength is gained in a hospital, it can operate at the supply chain level, from suppliers to patients receiving services, including Subdistrict Health Promoting Hospitals. This includes network connections for patient information flow, resource management such as drugs and medical supplies, and further information management and systems.

4.3.4 *Application of Barcodes in Hospital Logistics Systems*

Barcodes are used in various stages within hospitals, serving different objectives. Here are some of those practices:

1. This method is used for the identification of products during distribution. It can also be included on the Kanban card to record the usage amount in the system. This information is then used to replenish products or place orders. Points of use include the following:

    - Payment points at the depot.
    - Payment points at the OPD, with records sent to the warehouse.
    - Dispensing point at the IPD, with records sent to the central stock.

2. This method is used to identify products during the receiving process, reducing the steps of counting products and recording data into the system as illustrated in Figures 4.4 and 4.5. Points of use include the following:

    - Drug pick-up point.
    - Point for receiving medicines into central stock.

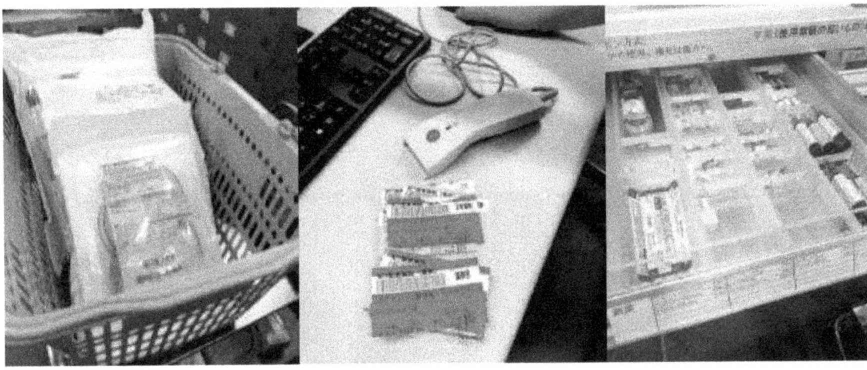

Figure 4.4. A barcode is attached to the product and the Kanban card. Scan each to record the transaction. After recording, return the Kanban card to pick up the product. There is also a barcode on the IPD medicine to be dispensed.

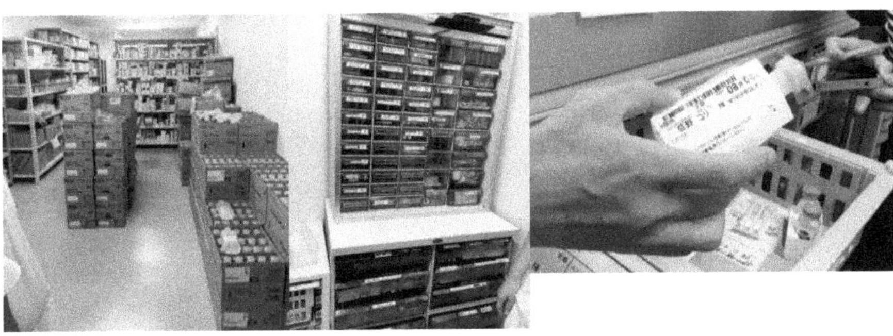

Figure 4.5. A barcode is attached to the package, which is scanned upon arrival at the IPD stock warehouse. This barcode is used to organize the one-day dose based on the doctor's prescription.

- Point for receiving medicines into IPD stock.
- One-day dose administration.

3. This specification is used to determine the storage location for products within the warehouse as shown in Figure 4.6.
4. It can be used for verifying the count and types of products, as shown in Figure 4.7.
   Points of use include:

- CSSD (Central Sterile Supply Department)

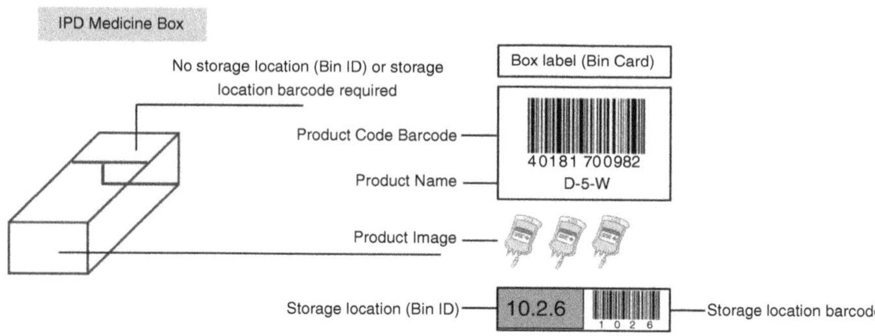

Figure 4.6. Barcodes are also used to pinpoint the storage location for products in the warehouse.

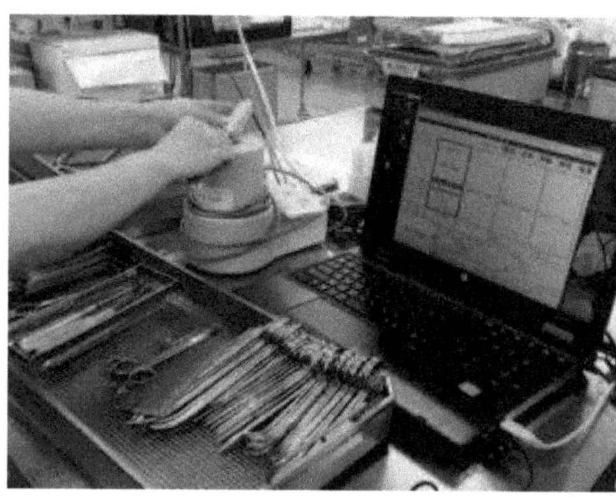

Figure 4.7. 2D barcodes are used to tally products and their types.

5. It can be used for entering patient identification, status, and history into the electronic medical records system (Figure 4.8).
6. Barcodes are used to identify products and evaluate their impact on patient safety during dispensing. A barcode is scanned to verify the patient identification number, product code (Figure 4.9), and operator code (Figure 4.10), confirming the product's dispensing to the patient.

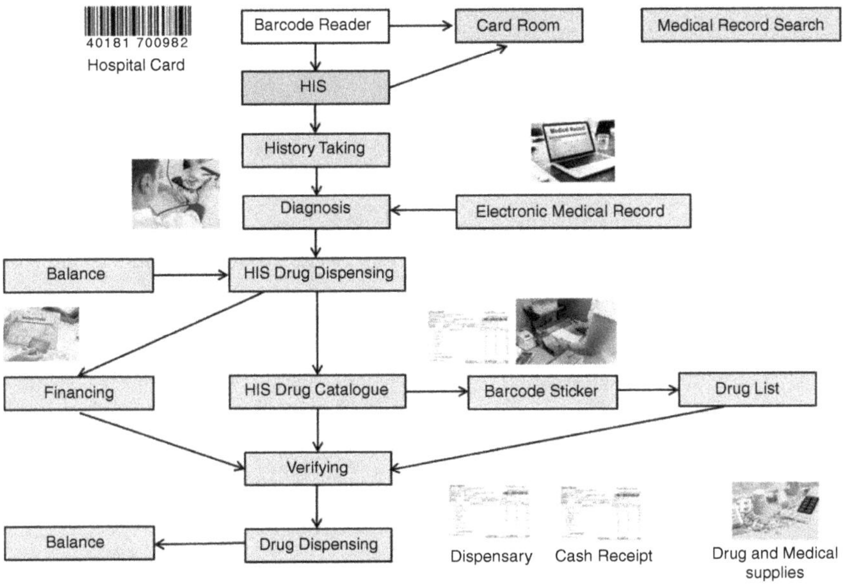

Figure 4.8. Barcodes are utilized to identify patient status and history within the system.

Note: HIS stands for Hospital Information System.

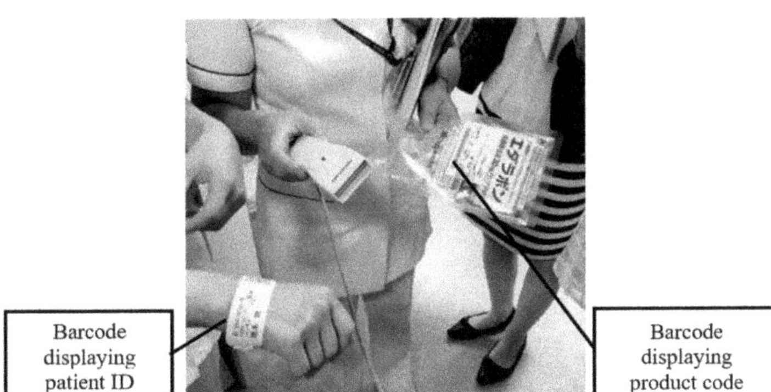

Figure 4.9. Scanning the barcode on the patient identification number and product code.

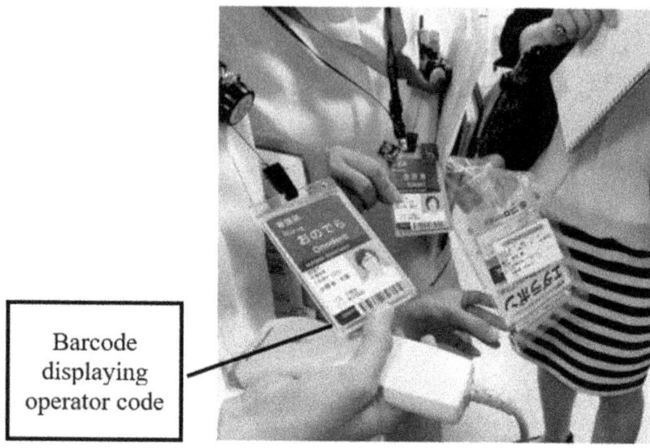

Figure 4.10. Scanning the barcode on the operator ID.

4.4 Conclusion

Improving hospital logistics requires more than isolated fixes; it demands structured action plans. This chapter outlined how hospitals can move from assessment and planning to design, execution, and evaluation. Examples illustrated the importance of standardizing processes such as procurement, warehousing, and electronic data exchange to build resilience and reduce fragmentation. Action plans provide a roadmap that aligns resources and activities with strategic goals.

The lessons learned from this chapter stress the importance of clear roles, responsibilities, and timelines. Without these, even the most well-designed plan is unlikely to succeed. Hospitals should aim to achieve quick wins, such as streamlining ordering systems, while also laying the groundwork for long-term transformation. Action plans that combine short-term improvements with strategic investments create sustainable change, ensuring that logistics systems can adapt to future challenges.

Chapter 5

Building Robust Logistics Infrastructure in Public Health System

5.1 Study of Design and Development for Logistics Infrastructure and Integrated Information System and Guidelines of Healthcare Big Data for Thailand Digital Economy Project

From a survey of Thailand's health expenditure accounts during 2009–2010 by the Strategy Office, the Ministry of Public Health found that the proportion of health expenditures for Thai people overall is quite stable, approximately 3.5–4.0% of gross domestic product (GDP), or equivalent to 392,368 million baht in health expenditures. However, when considering the proportion of expenditures on medicine, it was found that it had increased, especially for drugs outside the main drug list that are expensive. In addition, there are cases of smuggling and/or corruption of drugs and medical supplies that cannot be traced throughout the drug and medical supply chain. This makes it impossible to find the true cause and understand the situation. **The main reason is that Thailand lacks a standard data structure and a system for linking and exchanging information between members of the entire health supply chain. This includes the absence of a surveillance system and a lack of data for supervision, follow-up, and inspection of the efficient management of medicines and medical supplies. Although it is accurate and reliable, it is widely**

acknowledged at both the organizational and national levels that it cannot effectively driver the digital economy in the contemporary era. System linkage requires the identification of drug codes for each of the diverse health care facilities. To be able to link data and display the results of data analysis on drugs and medical supplies, such as data on the movement of drugs and medical supplies, quantity of medicines, and medical supplies received and dispensed in the health care facilities, so that central agencies can process such information for the benefit of health management services, decision support, and to determine health policy at the national level.

Research studies on logistics management at the health supply chain of Mahidol University, including the format for exchanging drug information in the public health supply chain for the safety and good health of public health service recipients (Kritchanchai *et al.* 2011–2013). The project is to develop a national drug database and an efficient internet search system and improve the safety of people's drug use, the pilot development of the use of Vendor Managed Inventory (VMI)/Electronic Data Interchange (EDI) principles for drugs and medical supplies (Kritchanchai *et al.*, Mahidol University and the Office of the Higher Education Commission 2011–2013) and the book on research cluster on logistics systems for improving the level of health and hygiene services in Thailand, Mahidol University. It was found that basic information (foundation), such as standard drug code formats, hospital supply chain business processes, data linking format and related information, business processes for electronic data exchange for health supply chains, including information used in exchange. These can serve as guidelines for developing a drug and medical supply inventory management system and leading to readiness for the digital economy.

The management of medicines, medical supplies, and other health products is crucial in helping reduce a country's expenses. One of the primary reasons for high administrative costs is the mutually exclusive manner in which management is conducted. There is a lack of integration and basic infrastructure for standards and data integration. Thailand's public health stakeholders consist of numerous agencies.

Logistics management systems, medicines, and medical supplies play a key role in the development of the country's public health system, necessitating urgent action. Any delay may negatively impact patient trust in the country's drug management system, as seen with Pseudoephedrine, illegally used as a precursor in the production of Amphetamine, which contains chemical compounds we in illicit drug production. Therefore, this project urgently prioritizes recruiting experts with specialized expertise in both information technology systems and drug and medical supply storage systems. The goal is to develop information and management systems for drugs and medical supplies, ensuring effective drug management, reducing costs in managing drug stocks, efficiently tracing system issues, preventing national-level problems and damages, and reducing errors due to expired or substandard medicines.

Therefore, the research team plans to undertake a project to develop a system for managing drug and medical supply inventory throughout the supply chain. **This project will apply findings from past studies in health logistics, conducted by the National Research Council of Thailand (NRCT) and the Thailand Research Fund (TRF) between 2013 and 2016.** The research aims to design and develop various work systems as follows:

Phase 1, Year 2016:

Ph. 1.1 Develop a drug and medical supply database system (National Medicinal Product Catalog Database: NMPCD) that can support linking and exchanging information with various related logistics agencies in the future.

Ph. 1.1 Design and develop a drug and medical supply warehouse management system (Material Management Information System: MMIS).

Phase 2, Year 2017:

Ph. 2.1 Develop an information and communication technology system master plan for the country's public health sector.

Ph. 2.2 Create a management program and prepare drug information for the Patient Information Leaflet Management System, including creating a drug store management program to link with the drug and medical supply database system.

Ph. 2.3 Develop standards for the medicine and medical supply management system (MMIS) and create manuals for application in various health service facilities in the country.

Ph. 2.4 Develop an electronic data interchange (EDI) system.
Ph. 2.5 Develop a tracking and traceability system for pharmaceutical logistics in Thailand (Traceability).

Phase 3, Year 2018:

Ph. 3.1 Develop an in-depth information system on medicines and medical supplies in hospitals under the Ministry of Public Health to support the strategic planning of medicines and medical supplies of the Ministry of Public Health (Business Intelligence: BI).
Ph. 3.2 Create the NMPCD system to connect with the public health service system and develop drug code standards for the Identification of Medicinal Products (IDMP).
Ph. 3.3 Create a connection system between the drug and medical supply inventory management system (Material Management Information System: MMIS) and the hospital's in-depth information system for drugs and medical supplies (BI) and related hospital internal systems to support the health information system of the Ministry of Public Health (Unified Health Data Platform).
Ph. 3.4 Study and develop the exchange and integration of electronic public health data for hospitals to lead to in-depth public health information processing in Thailand.

The concept framework for the entire system is shown in Figure 5.1.

e-Health Master Plan Healthcare Logistics

The challenge for collaborative management is integrating data and information on the same infrastructure (platform), linking data for management using shared information in both the public and private sectors, the industrial sector, and the education sector. It is a platform that can facilitate business operations together.

This project is, therefore, considered an important cooperation project in both Information and Communication Technology (ICT) and public health, the education sector, and the industrial business sector.

In 2016, a team of researchers (Duangpun *et al.*, 2016) conducted a study and developed a drug and medical supply database system. It can support recording data sets used in the health supply chain and designing data architectures in the health supply chain, including

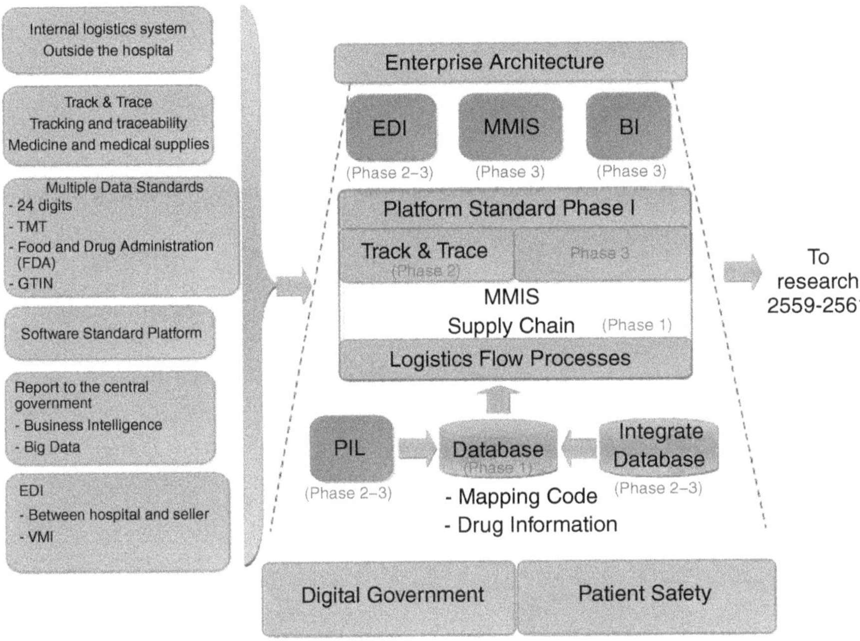

Figure 5.1. Conceptual framework for research.

developing roadmaps for drug codes that can be used throughout the system. It is an appropriate method for improving and developing communication models in the public health supply chain.

When considering the logistics system and supply chain within the hospital, it was found that the basic assumptions of the management of drug and medical supply warehouses in health administrative centers were found to be the results of interviews with 10 hospitals in the research project to develop the logistics system. Community hospital logistics (Duangpun *et al.*, 2015) and model hospitals in the project to apply logistics systems for the safety of service recipients in the primary hospital network system (Duangpun *et al.*, 2015) found that the hospital's MMIS is currently a standalone system, that is, there is no link to any data. With the patient service system (Front Office), important capabilities are recording receipts, payments, and counting product balances only.

The hospital inventory management system supports the condition of a single warehouse as shown in Figure 5.2. That is, when the goods have been dispatched from the main warehouse. Even if a

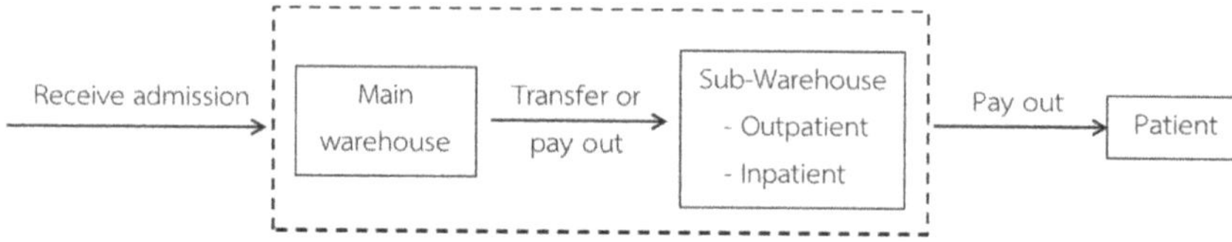

Figure 5.2. Hospital inventory management.

product is in use or has not yet been used by a patient, it will not be possible to check the overall balance of the hospital.

The inventory image in the MMIS system displays the balance of products stored in the main warehouse. However, it does not show the quantity of products at various sub-warehouses. There are certain limitations in the MMIS system as described above, impacting the operational efficiency. To improve this, the MMIS system should be adjusted in the following ways.

- The MMIS system should support a multi-warehouse model, enabling visibility of product balances in all warehouses, including the main warehouse, subdepots, and drug distribution points within the hospital.
- The display should indicate whether each storage warehouse will display the usage amount immediately (Nettable Inventory), helping the hospital to understand the remaining balance in various storage warehouses and plan, estimate, and purchase products more efficiently.
- The MMIS system should be capable of checking receipts and handling payments for products at the level of their trade name or brand.
- It should also support receiving and disbursing at the pack size level of the product to enable traceability and promote safety in medicine use.
- Lastly, the MMIS system should be linked with the patient service system to correctly and completely collect the total usage amount. This will reduce the workload of operators who must record duplicate data. The workflow of an appropriate MMIS system is shown in Figure 5.3.

National standards for medicine codes represent another significant issue. These codes are used and referenced throughout the supply chain, from registering drug formulas and purchasing drugs

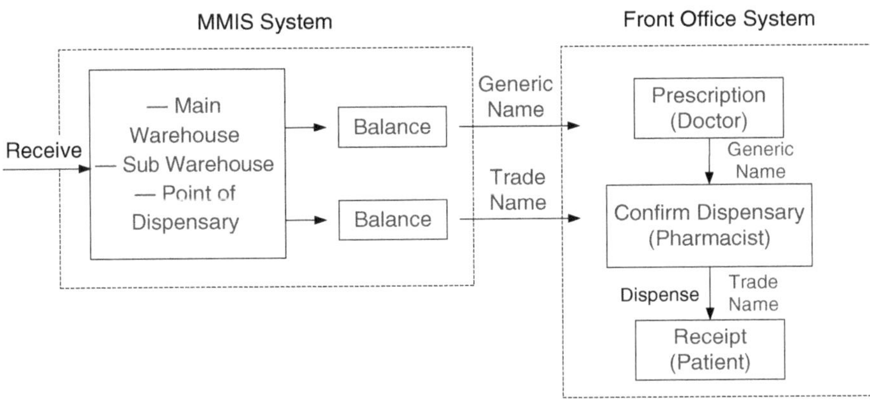

Figure 5.3. Appropriate MMIS system in a hospital.

to providing drug services and disbursing drug expenses. The specific code used varies.

Currently, there are four main codes for ready-made medicines in the health supply chain system:

1. Drug registration numbers are used to identify drug formulas submitted for registration for production or distribution in Thailand (Drug Act B.E. 2510).
2. The 24-digit drug code is designed to transmit drug usage data in the purchasing data section. This data is used to establish reference prices and information on inpatient orders in accordance with the 43 file standards. It also serves as information for monitoring drug indicator groups, including data for generating reports on current adverse drug reactions (spontaneous ADR) and has been in use since 1986.
3. TMT is used for disbursement and collecting statistical data on drug use and has been in use since 2013.
4. GTIN is used to identify products at the packaging level and has been in use since 1988.

Each drug code is used in the drug and medical supply chain process. Government agencies establish codes to serve the objectives of each department. However, there is no central database for collecting drug information. Each agency that issues codes maintains its own database, and the data items vary. There are no clear standards

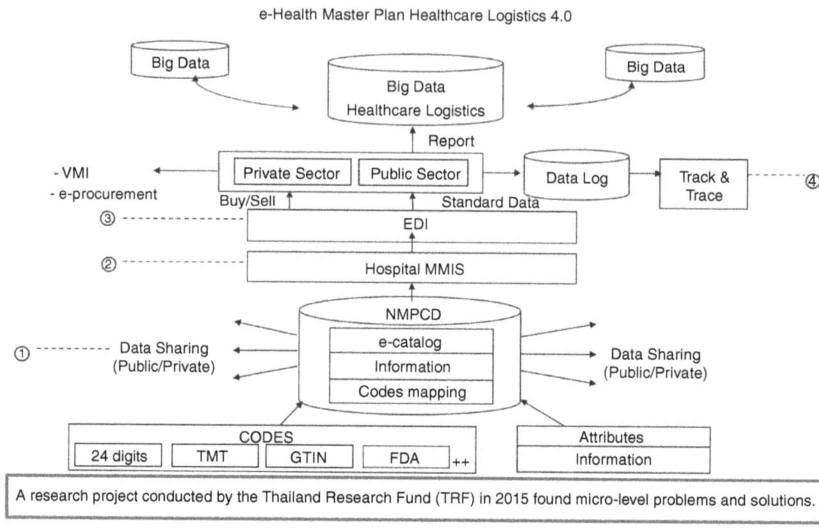

Figure 5.4. Conceptual framework for conducting research throughout the plan.

for data exchange or data linking. In addition, there is no logistics information on drug use that can be employed in health analysis and management, such as the quantity and reasonableness of use of drugs or medical supplies nationwide. It remains unclear what proportion of medicine is prescribed by doctors, nurses, or pharmacists or chosen by the patients themselves. Therefore, each code serves a different purpose, and no party is willing to standardize the code. Figure 5.4 illustrates how the research team carries out its operations.

5.1.1 *Phase 1, Year 2016*

(1) Ph. 1.1 National Medicinal Product Catalog Database (NMPCD): Develop a database system that compiles information and characteristics of drugs and medical supplies available in Thailand. The system will harmonize codes from various databases in Thailand and create a centralized database. This approach will make it easier for all departments to use and will also help reduce time and errors in data entry and drug code verification.

(2) Ph. 1.2 Material Management Information System (MMIS): Develop an inventory management program for drugs and medical supplies in hospitals. The MMIS research team will create a warehouse management system, ready for integration with NMPCD, and will include features used in logistics to reduce inventory and provide electronic data tracking.

The MMIS system will facilitate the management of drug and medical supply inventory within the hospital. It will allow visibility of inventory levels at the hospital's service points, enabling efficient warehouse management.

5.1.2 *Phase 2, Year 2017*

(3) Ph. 2.1 Development of an Information and Communication Technology System Master Plan for the Country's Public Health Sector: The goal is to develop a master plan and architecture for the country's information technology system. This will set the direction for development and drive strategy implementation. It can serve as a blueprint for creating various necessary systems for the country.

(4) Ph. 2.2 Program to Manage and Create Drug Information for the Public: This program aims to meet the basic needs of the people and maintain standards according to the process of developing drug information documents for the public. The documents will be linked to data on the business architecture of hospitals, drug stores, standard drug codes, and public health database structure standards.

(5) Ph. 2.3 Expanding Research on Material Management Information System (MMIS), Year 2016, to a Wider Circle: The aim is to expand the use of the drug and medical supply inventory management system in 10 health service facilities to improve efficiency and coverage. The MMIS system will be enhanced to link data between the drug and medical supply inventory management system in health service facilities and drug dispensing points in the health service facility's work system.

(6) Ph. 2.4 Electronic Data Exchange System (Electronic Data Interchange (EDI)): This system is used to exchange information electronically between the health service facilities of the Ministry of Public Health and various agencies such as the Comptroller General's Department and the Government Pharmaceutical Organization, and the Food and Drug Administration.

(7) Ph. 2.5 Drug and Medical Supply Tracking and Tracing System (Traceability): This system is designed to track and inspect the use of medicines and medical supplies in the facility, supporting inspections from the purchasing process to the hospital and patient level.

Theory, Hypothesis, and/or Conceptual Framework of the Research Plan: Drawing from the research project on logistics and health supply chains of the National Research Council of Thailand (NRCT) and the Thailand Research Fund (TRF) for 2013–2015, and research funds for policy response research plans/government goals for 2016 by the NRCT, the Ministry of Public Health, and the Hospital Pharmacy Association (Thailand), the conceptual framework for 2017 is divided into five subprojects:

1. Development of an information and communication technology system master plan for the country's public health sector.
2. Program for managing and creating drug information for the public.
3. Expanding the results of MMIS system research conducted in 2016 to a wider audience.
4. Electronic data exchange system.
5. Developing a tracking and traceability system for pharmaceutical logistics in Thailand (Traceability).

The details of these subprojects are as follows:

(1) Development of Information and Communication Technology System Master Plan for the Country's Public Health Sector: Health service systems generally encompass four main areas: medical treatment, disease prevention and control, health promotion services, and rehabilitation services. Health service work is interdisciplinary, involving communication with individuals from various occupations. Data management is important, as is communication between service professionals, providers, and recipients. Thailand organizes its healthcare system in stages, with a referral system for health services that range from basic primary care to complex tertiary and super-tertiary care:

1. Primary Health Services (Primary Care)
2. Secondary Health Services (Secondary Care)

3. Tertiary Health Services (Tertiary Care)
4. Health Services at a Level Higher than Tertiary (Super-Tertiary Care)

Thailand is one of the few countries worldwide with a universal health coverage system, with three main agencies managing its healthcare funds: the Office of Universal Health Coverage, the Comptroller General's Department (which looks after medical benefits for civil servants and their families), and the Social Security Office. The different payment methods and processes for these three health insurances challenge the development of a unified information system. Therefore, the design of the national health information must consider health financial mechanisms and the country's health service system.

Health and public health information systems are vital components of an efficient health system, especially health information systems. The health service system and health finance system must interact closely with each other. A subsystem's design must consider interconnected systems, and it is not possible to design a subsystem without considering other systems. Therefore, the development of the Health Information Technology system must be considered alongside the health finance system (Health Care Financing) and the health service system (Health Care Delivery). All three systems are closely linked and influence each other. Hence, the development of health information systems aligns with the context of the health service system and the country's health financial and fiscal mechanisms, divided into three levels of health information systems as shown in Figure 5.5.

1. Operational or Transactional Information Systems, such as health center service information systems or outpatient services in hospitals, support the work and decision-making of operators such as doctors, nurses, and health center staff at the point of medical care or service (Point of Care).
2. Management Information Systems are designed to assist managerial decision-making for department heads or hospital administrators. These systems draw on data from operational systems to inform decisions at the management level.
3. Executive Information Systems are information systems designed to support executives in decision-making for corporate strategy

- Management information system for strategic planning and high-level decision making in regional and departmental agencies central ministry

---

- Information system for management services in service agencies such as hospitals, provincial public health offices, and mid-level departments

---

- Information systems provided in health centers
- Information system for outpatient services in hospitals
- Clinical information system

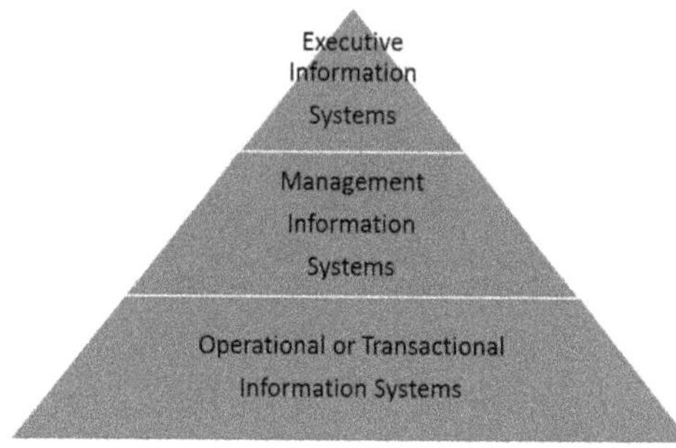

Figure 5.5. Components of health and public health information systems.

planning and high-level decisions. These systems have extensive data sources both inside and outside the organization. They manage lower-level information appropriately for executives who are tasked with making high-level decisions, not solving problems at the operational level.

To develop the country's health sector information and communication technology master plan for this research project, an integrated framework combining the Top Down and Bottom Up approaches was used. The Top Down approach sets the system structure from a broader, strategic planning perspective, while the Bottom Up Approach does so from the viewpoint of the system user or agency (micro perspective), as depicted in the following conceptual framework (Figure 5.6).

2. Develop a drug database system and create a program to manage and generate public drug information (Patient Information Leaflet Management System: PILMS): Upon reviewing the available drug information documents in Thailand, it appears that they can be categorized into different types as follows:

1. Medication package documents prepared by pharmaceutical companies for drug registration purposes. These documents contain information about every drug. This information is held by the Food and Drug Administration (FDA) and is distributed within a

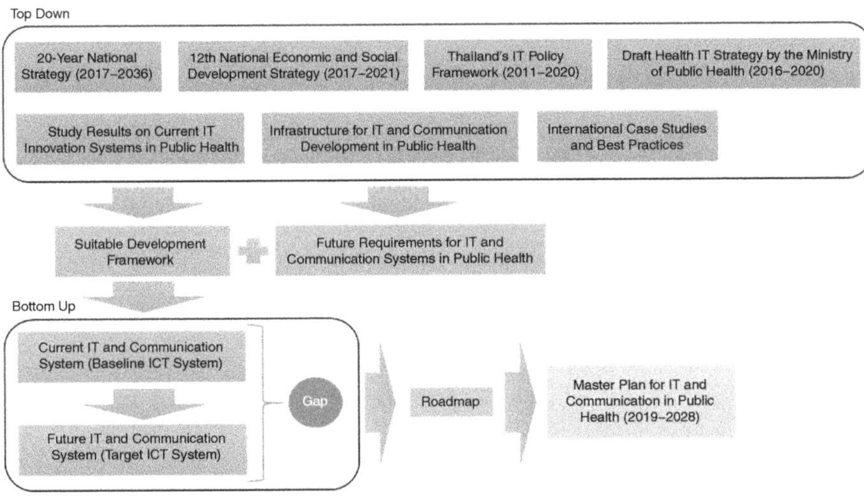

Figure 5.6. This is a conceptual framework for developing the master plan of the health sector's information and communication technology system.

limited circle. It exists in either electronic or physical format and can be found in each type of drug packaging.

2. Medication package documentation for medical personnel (SPC) is prepared by the FDA's working group, which includes faculty members from various pharmacy faculties. This group generates and reviews information from various primary sources, including Micromedex journals and other references. The information includes the product name, active ingredients, and their quantities. It describes the pharmaceutical characteristics and dosage forms of the drug. It outlines approved indications, recommended dosage, and methods of administration. Contraindications, warnings, and precautions are clearly specified. Potential drug–drug interactions and guidance for use in pregnant and lactating women are also provided. In addition, the information addresses effects on driving and operating machinery, possible adverse reactions, overdose management, and the drug's pharmacodynamic and pharmacokinetic properties.
3. The Prescription Indicator for Citizens (PIL) guidelines are prepared by the same committee as mentioned the point two. These guidelines assist in preparing drug documentation for the public, using various primary reference documents and Micromedex journals. The information provided, such as the purpose of the

medicine, usage instructions, and precautions, is less detailed than that in the second section. However, the amount of drug information available to the public is still relatively limited, due to a lack of experts in the field. The FDA working group has attempted to organize a workshop to disseminate guidelines for preparation in order to obtain more items in the second and third categories, but the amount of data is still low. The preparation of this drug control document is still done manually (Manual).
4. The drug package inserts provided by Ya&You are not very reliable, but they are widely available and contain more information on many medicines than other agencies' leaflets.
5. UHosNet provides supplementary medicine labels that include basic usage instructions, such as chewing the medicine thoroughly. However, these labels are not widely used and do not provide sufficient information given the current number of medicines available.

Therefore, the research team is interested in studying and developing a prototype system for creating a drug management program. This program would include drug information for the public, covering both modern human medicine and modern herbal medicine. The goal is to meet the public's basic needs and establish standards for developing drug information documents. This will involve cooperation from both the public and private sectors to maintain a consistent format, and the information will be applied to the Drug and Medical Supplies Database (NMPCD) system. This system will link drug information, including drug names, strengths, forms, and manufacturers and distributors, with the FDA-registered information to create a standard drug database for use in logistics systems. This information will be integrated into the drug and medical supply management program (MMIS) used in hospitals.

3. Expanding 2016 research findings to a broader audience: From the 2016 Phase 1 research project on designing and developing logistics systems, infrastructure, information integration systems, and Big Data initiatives for Thailand's digital economy in public health, the research team has designed an infrastructure system. This includes a hospital information system for managing drug and medical supply inventories. The system operates under the concept of an open platform, which allows anyone to use existing services for future program development (Figure 5.7).

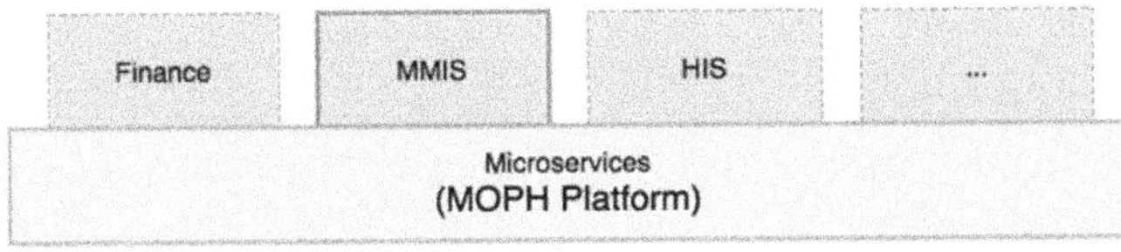

Figure 5.7. Concept of using microservices to create an open platform.

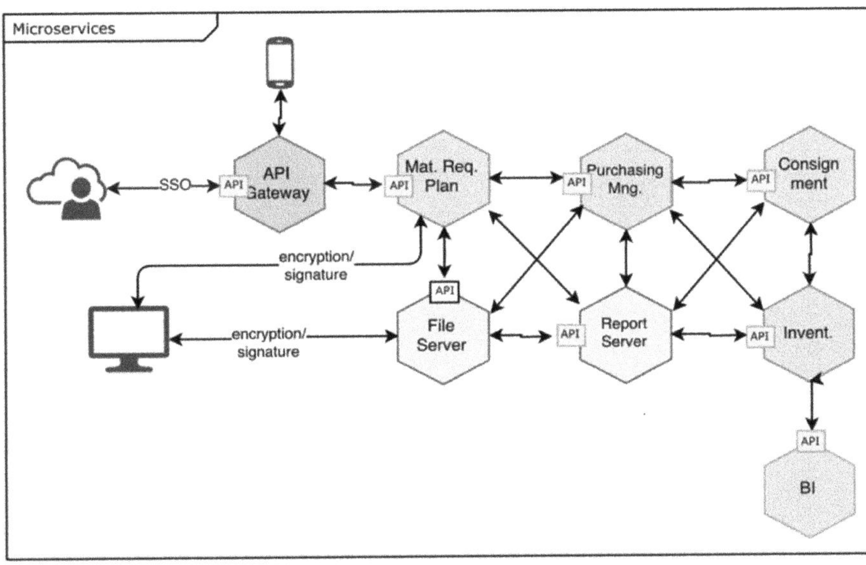

Figure 5.8. Structure of the medicine and medical supplies management system (MMIS).

From a study of drug and medical supply warehouse systems in various hospitals, including the examination of information systems for managing such warehouses, such as INV-C, INV-S, and so on, the research team designed the structure of microservices for the drug and medical supply management system. The design is illustrated in Figure 5.8. The research team designed various services for the drug and medical supply warehouse management system. Specifically, we created subservices for each group, particularly for the Main Section (Business Process) group and the Support Section group.

From Figure 5.9, in the Main Section, the MMIS program is designed to include a Decision Support System (DSS) as a separate group of services from the Material Requirements Planning (MRP)

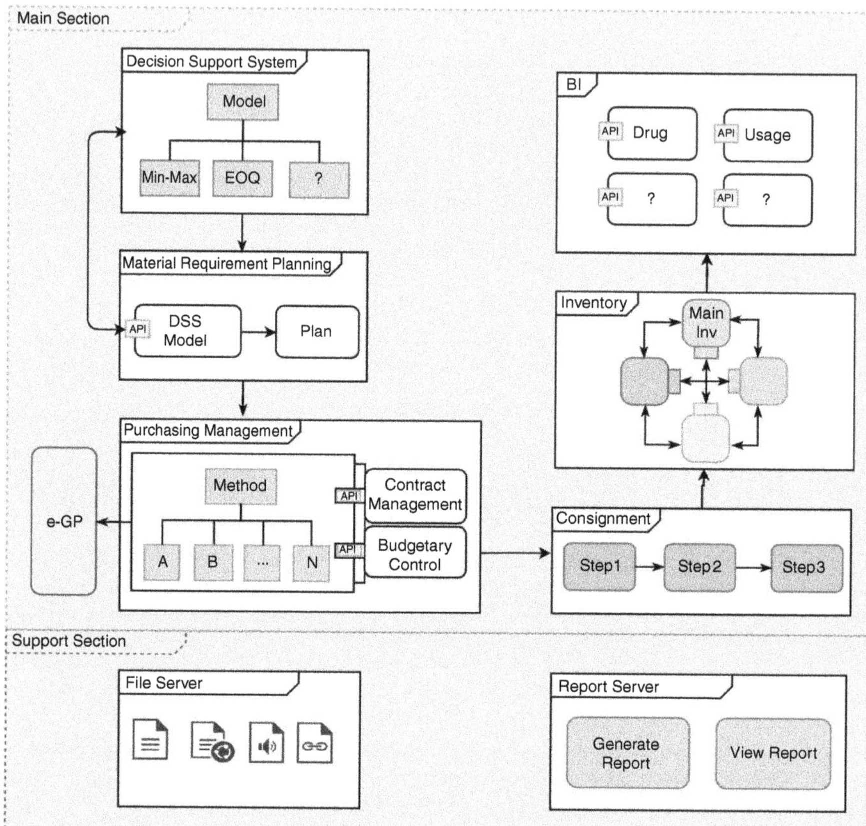

Figure 5.9. Service details in the MMIS system at the hospital.

system. This is because the DSS Service can be utilized in various ways and can support decision-making in other areas, such as planning for drug withdrawal from various warehouses. Therefore, the DSS Service involves the creation of subservices in the form of various models, such as Min-Max EOQ or other models, to support decision-making in various types of work.

In the Inventory Service, each warehouse in the hospital is a group of services that can be independently linked to other warehouses. This is because each hospital has a different structure of the main drug warehouse and subdrug warehouses. However, if we view each drug warehouse as merely a group of services that work together, we can create a drug warehouse structure independently according to the needs of each hospital.

In the BI Service, it is similar to the DSS Service in terms of creating a model to summarize information for executives. This allows developers to further develop BI in various forms by integrating additional services into the BI Service.

Finally, every system can access the Support Service, which currently comprises two groups: file servers and report servers. These manage documents and various types of reports within the hospital. Separating the services in the Support group allows other systems, in addition to the MMIS system, to utilize these services. This will enable each hospital to develop its own information system more conveniently and quickly.

The research study on healthcare supply chain logistics management at Mahidol University highlighted the crucial role of managing medicines, medical supplies, and other health products in cutting down the country's costs. One primary reason for the escalated management costs is the disjointed and non-integrated nature of management, coupled with a lack of standardized infrastructure and data integration. Therefore, it is suggested to broaden the system development for managing the warehouse of medicines and medical supplies in healthcare facilities. This expansion could bolster the Thai public health system and prepare it for the digital economy.

4. Electronic data interchange (EDI) system: Efficiency in a health supply chain's logistics process is necessary for improving safety and service provision in healthcare. It allows for traceability and resolves issues related to medication storage errors, counterfeit products, and product recalls. A study of the information technology systems used within hospitals and distributors revealed a variety of systems in use. This diversity can cause problems in electronic data exchange between hospitals and distributors, resulting in work redundancy, process delays, and unnecessary paperwork-related expenses. To mitigate these issues, the EDI system has been introduced to manage the health supply chain in Thailand.

The EDI system is a platform that transmits data electronically between organizations, aiming to increase efficiency in commercial operations.

EDI is a component of electronic commerce (E-Commerce) that exchanges standard structured data between computers via electronic means. This structured data is transmitted over the Internet, enabling data to be sent or retrieved for processing. EDI involves the computer-to-computer exchange of information using electronic documents as the medium. These documents, used to send and receive information, must be in a standard format approved by both the recipient and the sender. Such electronic documents can be transmitted through both parties' computer systems without the need for paper printing.

When exchanging information electronically, three elements should be considered, as follows:

1. The EDI software application is designed to convert received messages into basic data formats used internally by an organization, and vice versa. This allows messages from partner companies to flow directly into the application. Software selection should be made considering not only the need for connectivity with other information systems but also relevant business and technical considerations.
2. The EDI standards structure the data in documents that organizations use for trade, such as product codes, product lists, prices, and addresses. This standard consists of rules specifying how to design the message for exchange. Examples of commonly used EDI standards are as follows:
    - ANSI X.12 (American National Standard Institute X12) is a main standard in North America and is widely used in Australia and New Zealand.
    - UN TDI (United Nations Trade Data Interchange) is a main standard in Western Europe and is extensively used in England as a component of TRADACOMS.
    - EDIFACT (Electronic Data Interchange for Administration, Commerce, and Transport) is an international standard that is currently the most popular in the business world because business transportation and services are not limited to within the country or region.
    - ebXML (Electronic Business Extensible Markup Language) is a collaboration between the UN/CEFACT agency, controlled by the United Nations, and OASIS, a non-profit organization

formed by the merger of information technology companies. This collaboration created an open standard that is internationally accepted. It uses the principles of XML to help specify the structure of the data and is announced as the ISO/DTS 15000:2004 standard.

3. Electronic communication structures enable swift information flow between partner companies. The EDI Network or Value-Added Network (VAN) service providers function as communication channels. The VAN service providers can be categorized into two main types: (1) domestic VAN service providers, with service centers in Thailand, primarily providing network services within the country, and (2) international EDI service providers, with service centers located abroad, mainly serving international networks.

A study of hospital business processes revealed that information is conveyed between hospitals and distributors in various formats. Many still rely on paper documents to issue purchase orders, which are sent to distributors via fax or email. The current ordering process in hospitals begins with officials checking the drug warehouse to determine if it is time to reorder. They then issue a purchase request (PR) and send it to the distributor to check product availability. This PR is also sent to the purchasing department to issue a Purchase Order (PO), which is then authorized and sent to the distributor for confirmation. The distributor sends the products, along with a delivery order (DO) and invoice, to the hospital's warehouse department. Officials inspect, receive, and store the medicines and medical supplies in the warehouse. They create a Goods Received Note (GRN) to record the receipt of goods and confirm their delivery. The GRN is a crucial document that the finance department uses to cross-reference with the PO and invoice before making payment.

Given that most data are manually transmitted via paper (Figure 5.10), there is a high potential for errors in communication, leading to time and cost inefficiencies. Therefore, the use of an Electronic Data Interchange (EDI) system in hospitals could be a big improvement.

Studies and research from the Center of Excellence in Health Supply Chain Management at Mahidol University have presented a prototype of the EDI/VMI program. This system, running on a cloud

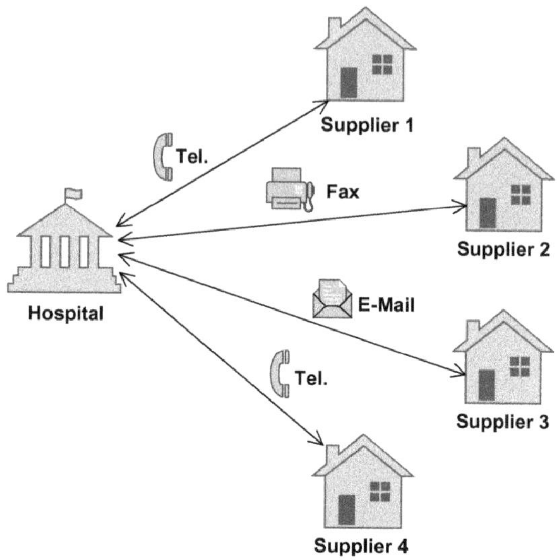

Figure 5.10. Manual process for transmitting order data in the hospital.

server, consists of a database server and application server or is sent through a Value-Added Network (VAN) that supports data exchange between hospitals and distributors via the internet. The ordering process through the EDI system starts with the purchasing department issuing a PO in the hospital system and sending it to the EDI Portal for the distributors. Once the distributor receives the PO, they inspect the products and schedule a delivery date. Before delivering the products, an advance shipment notice (ASN) document is sent to the hospital to provide details about the product and the scheduled delivery date. Upon receiving the ASN and after product inspection, the information in the ASN can be entered into the hospital system. This allows officials to know the product details and related purchase orders, significantly reducing the time it takes to receive products into the hospital warehouse in Figure 5.11.

The electronic data exchange process within the hospital begins with the ordering process. This encompasses purchase management, shipping, calling for payment for goods, and the payment of goods. Each process has documented information on deliveries. The main documents include PO, ASN, and invoices for electronic data exchange in hospital supply chains. After organizing small

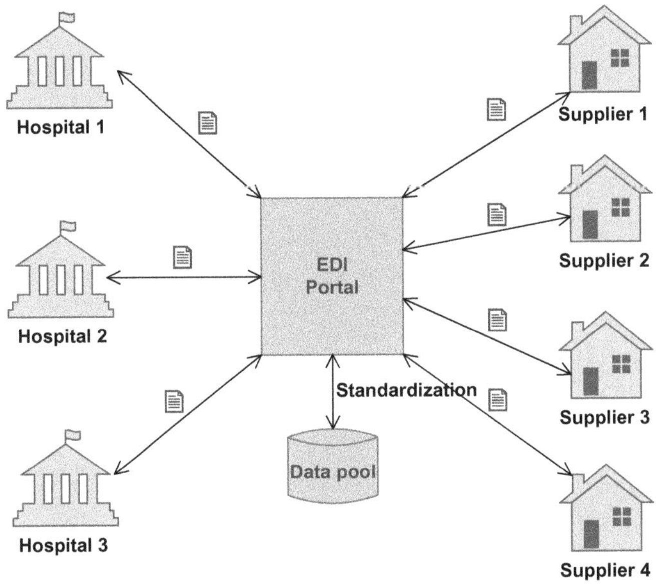

Figure 5.11. Process of EDI order data transmission.

group meetings and reaching an agreement between relevant agencies, both tertiary hospitals and distributors concluded on a pilot system for electronic data exchange in hospital supply chains. This system focuses on PO and ASN, with a data set of these documents obtained from a joint summary between the hospital and the supplier.

A study on the information technology systems used within hospitals and distributors revealed a variety of systems in use, and a lack of standards in information exchange between departments. Duplicate documents, delays, expenses, and wastage are frequent issues. To solve these problems, an electronic data exchange system or EDI should be implemented to exchange information and documents between hospitals and drug and medical supply distributors. This system could reduce errors that may occur in communication and delivery of purchasing documents. It will also improve tracking and traceability of drug and medical supply information, thereby increasing confidence in health services. A detailed comparison of the traditional manual processes versus the new EDI-enabled workflow in hospitals is summarized in Table 5.1.

Table 5.1. Comparison of old and new processes through EDI in hospitals.

Stakeholder	Original Process	EDI Process
Hospital	1. The purchasing department issues a Purchase Request (PR) and faxes it to the distributor to check product availability. 2. The purchasing department issues a Purchase Order (PO) in the hospital system. 3. The purchasing department faxes the PO to the distributor to confirm it. 4. The product inspection department inspects the products sent by the distributor along with the invoice. 5. The goods receiving department inspects the goods in the hospital system.	1. The purchasing department issues a PO in the hospital system. The system pulls the PO information into the EDI system and sends it to the distributor. 2. The product inspection department checks the receipt of goods sent by the distributor according to the Advance Shipping Notice (ASN) in the EDI system. 3. The goods receiving department inspects the goods in the hospital system. The system also pulls data into the EDI system.
Distributor	1. The sales department receives a PR form via fax from the hospital to check product availability. 2. The warehouse checks product quantity. 3. The sales department receives a PO via fax from the hospital. 4. The warehouse prepares products for delivery to the hospital. 5. The transportation department delivers the products to the hospital at the specified date and time.	1. The sales department enters the EDI system to confirm product quantity and creates an ASN document to notify the hospital of the product delivery date and time. 2. The warehouse prepares products for delivery to the hospital. 3. The transportation department delivers the products to the hospital at the specified date and time.

5. Development of a tracking and traceability system for drug logistics in Thailand (traceability): Patient safety is of significant medical importance. The World Health Organization (WHO) defines patient safety as minimizing the risks associated with health services, including those that should not occur, to an acceptable level (Walton *et al.*, WHO, Piyawan). Previous studies on hospital logistics management (McKinsey & Company, 2012; Duangpun, 2013) suggest that patient safety can be enhanced by preventing medication errors. These errors can arise from various factors, including the following:

1. Administering the wrong dosage, such as giving an incorrect concentration of medicine.
2. Administering medication to the wrong patient.
3. Administering incorrect medication as prescribed by the doctor, such as providing medicines that have deteriorated due to improper storage or are expired.
4. Administering medication at the wrong time, such as giving medicine before meals instead of after meals.
5. Administering medication through the wrong route, such as administering oral medication through a vein.

According to a report from the National Patient Safety Agency (NPSA) in 2007, almost 60,000 medication errors were identified between January 2005 and June 2006. The three most common types of errors were administering the wrong dose, administering medication at the wrong time, and incorrect medication administration as per the doctor's instructions. Together, these errors accounted for 57.3% of all reported mistakes, with the wrong dose being the most common issue, making up 28.7% of all reported errors (NPSA, 2007). These problems can be prevented through traceability, which allows for the following:

1. Verification during drug preparation and dispensing,
2. Tracking and tracing back to the origin of medications,
3. The ability to recall medicines if issues arise.

This tracking and tracing is applied throughout the supply chain (supply chain traceability). This means that if drugs or medical supplies flow through any system or process, they can be tracked and traced back.

Various activities in the health logistics system, from the manufacturer, distributors, hospitals, and patients, are interrelated with patient safety. Products produced and circulated through the system to the patient must be safe and free of contaminants. This is because medicine is consumed by patients, enters the body, and directly impacts health and life.

The ability to track and trace the supply chain of medicines and medical supplies (supply chain traceability) helps enhance safety in providing medical treatment to patients. Tracking and traceability refer to the capability to follow (tracking) the movement of goods throughout logistics systems and supply chains. It also refers to tracing back to the history, application, or past location of items of interest, in this case, drugs and medical supplies (GS1, 2013). From this definition, it can be concluded that tracking and traceability consist of two critical steps: tracking and tracing, as illustrated in Figure 5.12.

If issues arise with products upon delivery, customers can trace them back to their source. This could be the production site or the origin of the raw materials used. This traceability allows us to pinpoint problem areas in the supply chain, whether they are with raw materials, production, storage, or transportation. As a result,

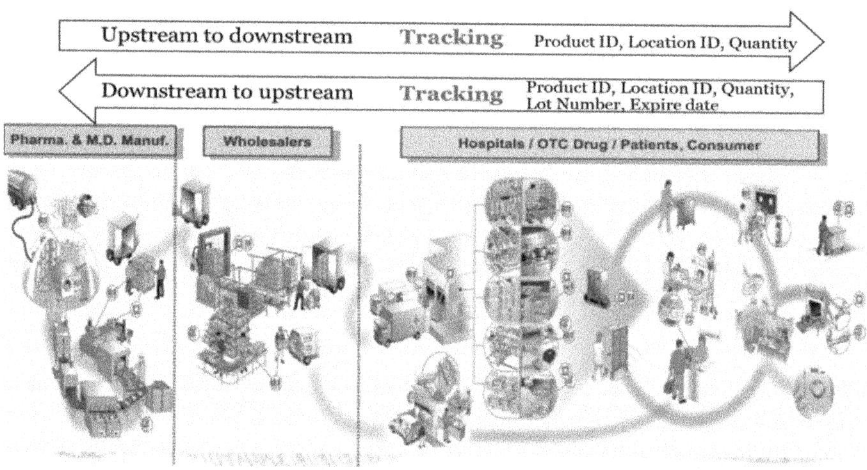

Figure 5.12. Product flow process in the public health supply chain and traceability.

Source: GS1 Japan, 2013.

the ability to track and trace drugs and medical supplies can substantially improve patient care by revealing the product's origin and production journey. If any issues warrant a recall of the drugs or medical supplies, they can be promptly addressed. This important concern is gaining more attention from manufacturers in Thailand (Chalermchan, 2010).

Primary hospitals, including community hospitals and Subdistrict Health Promoting Hospitals, currently face challenges in their logistics systems due to a lack of information linkage in the supply chain. This makes tracking and tracing drugs and medical supplies inefficient. Despite the critical role of tracking and tracing in patient safety, research and prototype system development have only recently begun, as indicated by a project on data traceability for efficient logistics and drug supply chain management. This has prompted research that leverages data from the hospital's business architecture, standard drug codes, public health database structure standards, and past tracking and traceability projects. The research aims to design data standards, databases, and supply chains to aid the implementation of a tracking system. This system is expected to enhance the efficiency of tracking and tracing drugs and medical supplies in hospitals, ultimately improving patient care and the quality of life for the Thai population.

6. Project case studies developing a COVID-19 vaccine cold chain to control temperature and traceability in transportation and storage: The research concept stems from the severity and rapid spread of the new 2019 coronavirus strain (COVID-19). Vaccines are viewed as a crucial solution to the COVID-19 outbreak in many countries, including Thailand. Plans are underway to import vaccines and expedite the vaccination of a large population to build herd immunity. The processes of importing and vaccinating are critical, especially given the short development time of these vaccines. There should be an effective tracking and tracing system to support these processes. Vaccine transportation relies on cold chain transportation to preserve the vaccine's effectiveness, a crucial step in delivering effective vaccines to the public. Considerable attention has been given to previous research and information technology systems, both domestically and internationally, concerning the traceability system in the health industry. In many countries, systems are developed to detect, evaluate, and prevent adverse events or other vaccine-related issues, including the prevention or reduction of vaccine falsification. Countries such as China, India, and Indonesia have faced significant counterfeiting issues, prompting government intervention. The government plays a key role in policy-making and enforcement, from the registration process to licensing. Many countries consider linking information with vaccination record systems for digital database storage. In Thailand, there is education and a tracking and traceability system, with data standards required for transmission in the health supply chain. However, there has been no design and development that covers the supply chain and can be applied in practice in this way before. Additionally, other information technology systems have not yet been developed to link and track the entire vaccine process, including where the vaccine was received, its origin, its status, where it was administered, and when it was given. In the past, Thailand has lacked an information system that can link and track the flow of vaccines and trace back vaccines in electronic form. Most vaccine data management systems and temperature controls are still separate and primarily use manual recording systems. Therefore, if a crisis such as this occurs, there should be a plan and development of a system to control and track vaccines at the national level.

From the above, it was found that there is a gap in research and development, including issues with temperature control during transportation. Each stage of vaccine delivery can affect the vaccine's effectiveness, as vaccines are biological materials sensitive to temperature changes. Vaccines can lose quality if exposed to inappropriate temperatures. Currently, service providers cannot monitor and track the vaccine's temperature during transportation in real time. Hence, if a batch of vaccines is compromised, it is unclear whether the issue is due to temperature fluctuations or the vaccine manufacturer. This is a concern for maintaining maximum patient safety. A comprehensive cold chain logistics system is crucial for vaccine providers. Vaccines providers need real-time access to shipment status throughout the entire delivery route to address issues promptly. Therefore, the COVID-19 Vaccine Cold Chain Traceability System's information flow was developed.

The research team has developed a cold chain tracking system for COVID-19 vaccines. This system tracks vaccines from upstream within the country (including importing agencies or manufacturing companies) to service providers (hospitals) and recipients of immunization service recipients. The emphasis is on creating tools that maximize efficiency and fit the current situation. The conceptual framework for this system is shown in Figure 5.13.

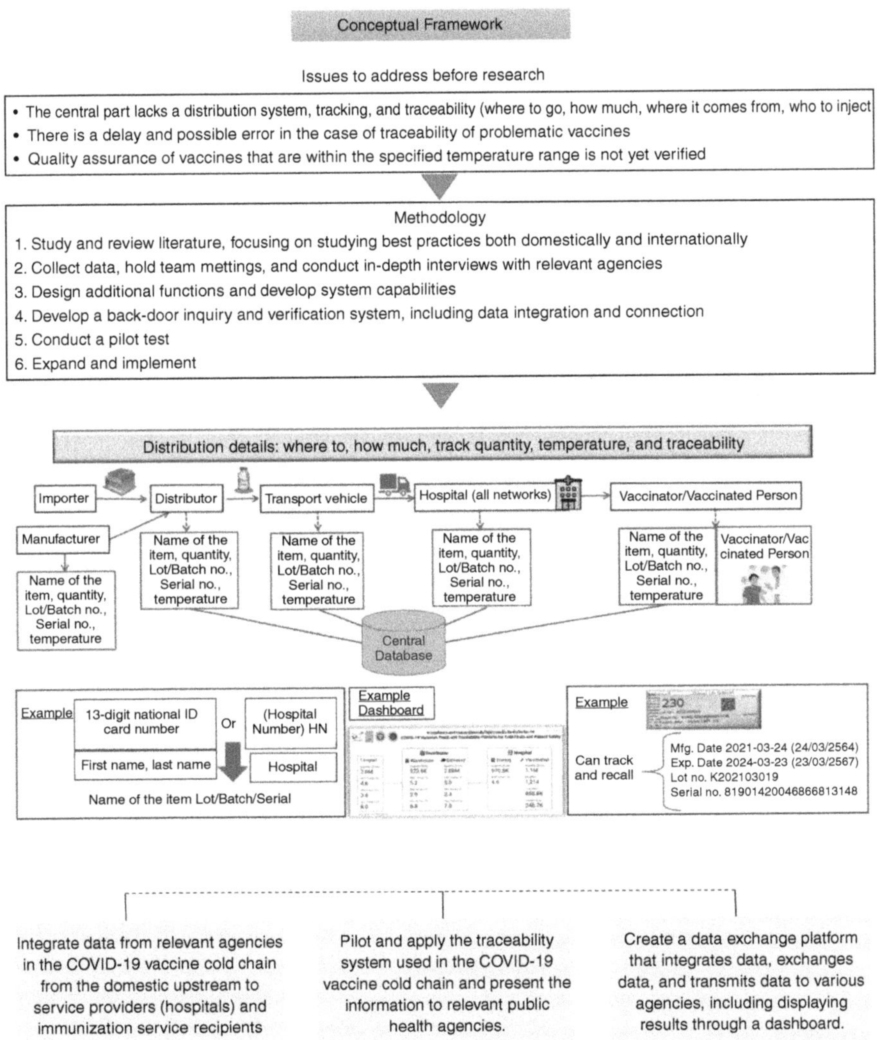

Figure 5.13. Research conceptual framework.

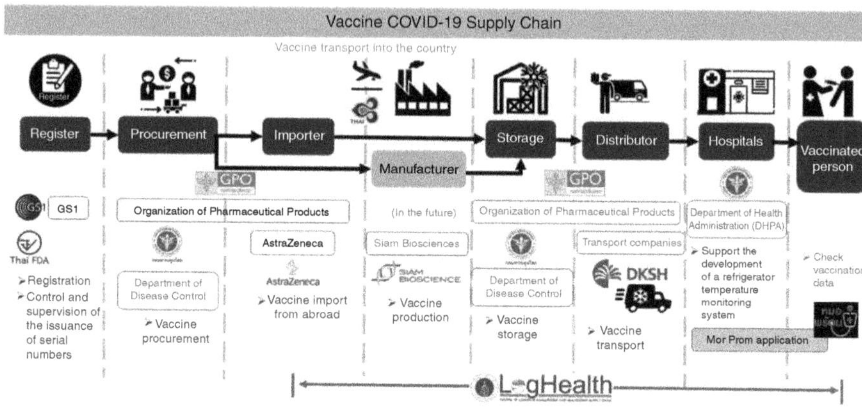

Figure 5.14. Current COVID-19 vaccine supply chain in Thailand.

Through a literature review, preliminary information gathering, and interviews with relevant individuals, the team has summarized the current COVID-19 vaccine supply chain in Thailand. This is illustrated in Figure 5.14.

Summary of data collection and in-depth interview results with relevant agencies for system design and expansion

From the collection of primary data and analysis of secondary data, it is evident that the agencies responsible for the COVID-19 vaccine control system in Thailand have the following roles and responsibilities as described in Table 5.2.

Figure 5.15 illustrates the process involving various relevant agencies (stakeholders) for determining important data sets and designing a comprehensive COVID-19 vaccine tracking and traceability system. The process begins with the import/production information. In this scenario, the Government Pharmaceutical Organization (GPO) engages a transport company to distribute vaccines to hospitals, which then transmit the information. Hence, the research team initiated a study of the process up to the point of administering the vaccines, as depicted in Figure 5.15.

By interviewing relevant agencies involved in the COVID-19 vaccine cold chain, the research team has summarized key data sets for system design, as detailed in Figure 5.16.

Table 5.2. Roles and duties of relevant agencies.

Agency	Roles and Duties
Food and Drug Administration (FDA)	Vaccine registration
Government Pharmaceutical Organization (GPO)	Purchasing, sourcing, and importing
Department of Medical Sciences	Production and import model certification (lot release)
Department of Disease Control (DDC)	Vaccine distribution plan creation
Distributor and Transport Companies	Transportation and distribution according to the vaccine distribution plan
Hospital	Receiving and storing vaccines for public injection
Subdistrict Health Promoting Hospital (client hospital) or outside hospital injection point	Receiving vaccines from the host hospital for public injection
Public Health Administration Division (P.H.A.D.)	Supervising and managing vaccine receipt, storage, and distribution to various hospitals
Information Technology Center, Ministry of Public Health	Receiving, storing, and forwarding information to relevant agencies
Nova Green and PTT ARV	Information related to vaccine temperature, storage, transportation, etc.
The Doctor is Ready	Overall vaccine information

The process begins with gathering needs through interviewing relevant agencies and conducting document analysis. This information is then used to design the functionality of the traceability system for the COVID-19 vaccine cold chain. The interactions between the system and the user in each use case are explained, and the insights gained from this requirement analysis are used in the next step. This includes designing the system functionality, architecture, and database system. The details are as follows.

5.1.3 *Functionality of the track and trace system*

In cases where there may be quality issues with the vaccine, such as suspected lapses in temperature control during transportation or

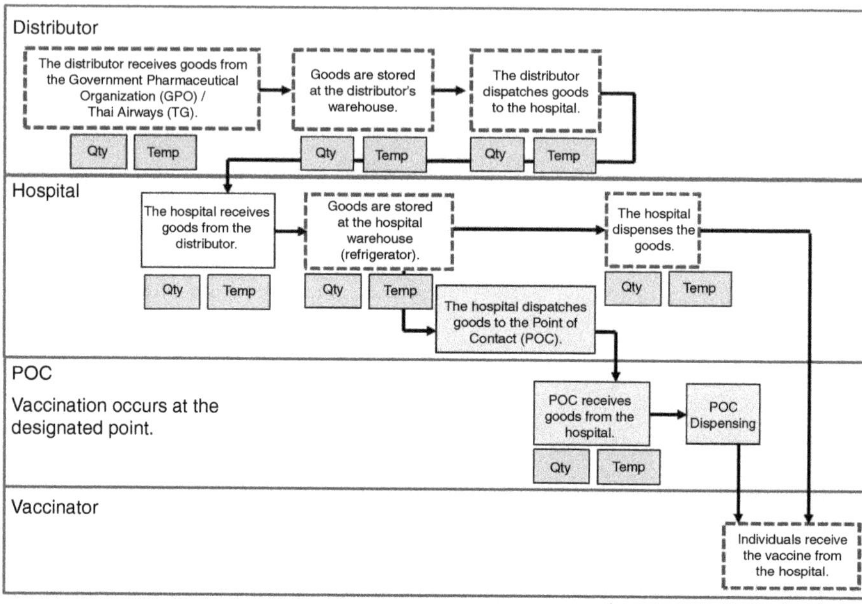

Figure 5.15. Framework for the flow of information and vaccines from upstream to downstream.

storage, a tracking and traceability system helps answer the following questions:

1. Which manufacturer produced the vaccine, and in which country?
2. Has the temperature been maintained as recommended by the manufacturer during transportation from the manufacturer to the storage area?
3. Is the storage temperature maintained as recommended by the manufacturer while waiting for distribution?
4. Is the temperature maintained as recommended by the manufacturer during transportation to a hospital or injection center?
5. Is the temperature maintained as recommended by the manufacturer during storage at hospitals or injection centers?

The responsibilities of the COVID-19 vaccine monitoring and traceability system are divided into seven parts:

1. Overview
2. Import/Manufacturer (import/production data)

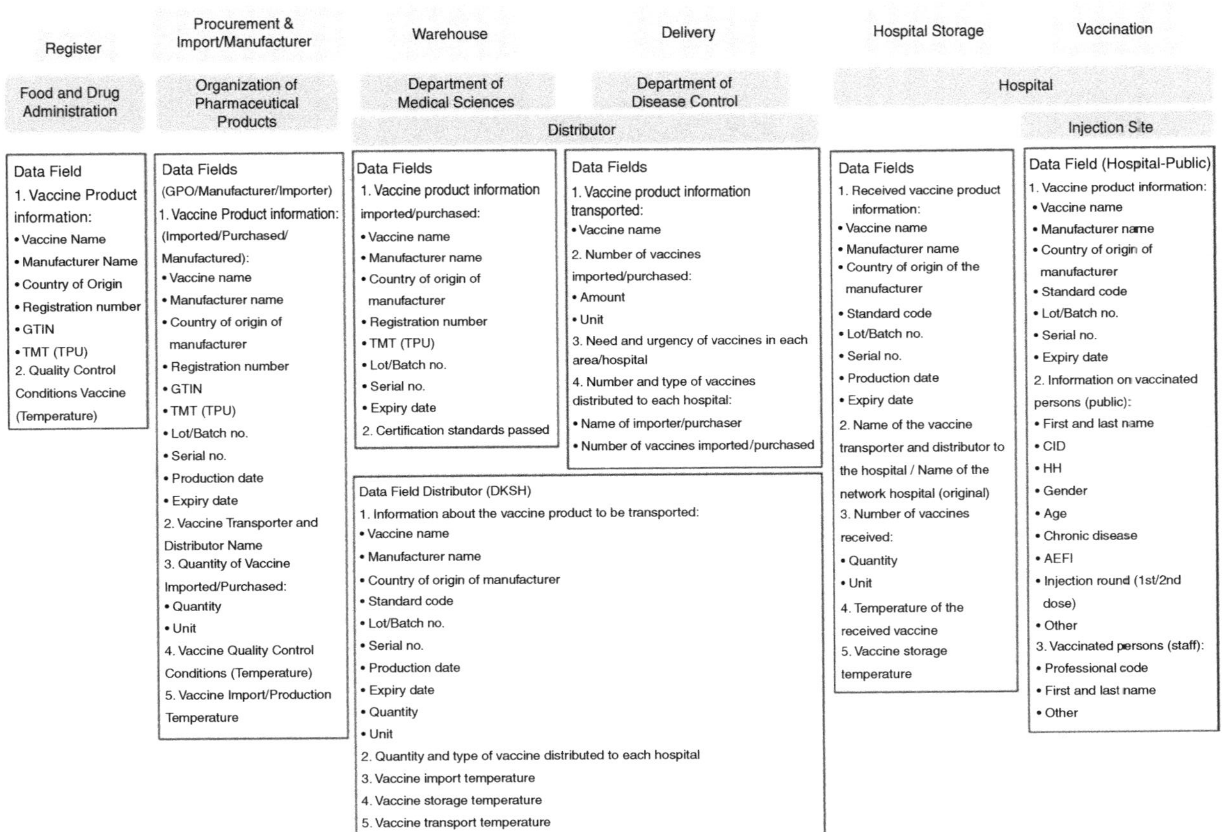

Figure 5.16. Key data sets for designing a COVID-19 vaccine tracking and traceability system.

3. Distributor (data at the distributor's warehouse and during transportation)
4. Delivery (vaccine distribution information)
5. Hospital (data about storage at the hospital warehouse)
6. Vaccination (injection information)
7. Serial (detailed product number information at the serial level)

The details are provided in Table 5.3.

5.1.4 *Research results*

The research project for cold chain development of COVID-19 vaccines aims to control temperature and ensure traceability during transportation and storage. The research team studied and reviewed literature, focusing on best practices both domestically and abroad. They collected data through meetings and in-depth interviews with relevant agencies to improve the cold chain traceability system used for the COVID-19 vaccine. The results of this research is a central platform that centralizes vaccine information. The system receives information from all agencies involved in the COVID-19 vaccine cold chain, from upstream within the country (importing agency or manufacturing company) to service providers (hospitals) and immunization recipients. Transport companies send information into the system through an SFTP Server developed by the team. This information includes import and distribution details. For hospitals and immunization service recipients, the system receives data through the Application Programming Interface (API) system. Data connections are divided into three types: temperature data connection (data from the IoT system, currently, temperature data from temperature measuring devices of two agencies are connected: PTT, ARV, and NOVA Green), vaccination data connection, and hospital vaccine movement data connection (movement) via the API of the Information Technology Center, Ministry of Public Health. The system will then process and display a vaccine data report (dashboard).

This system allows users to make use of information to address issues with vaccines at the batch, serial, and individual vaccination levels. It also provides information about vaccine distribution in each area, as well as data on each type of vaccination administered in these areas. The system has been in active use since 2021 and up

Table 5.3. Functions of the COVID-19 vaccine monitoring and traceability system.

Functions and Operation of the System	Details
1. Overview	• The system should display the following information on the minimum, maximum temperature, and MKT values: — Import/Production information — Data from distribution and transport companies' warehouses — Vaccine distribution information — Information stored at the hospital warehouse — Injection information
2. Import/ Manufacturer	• The system must display the total number of vaccines that have been imported or manufactured. • The system should provide the vaccine information every time it is imported or produced, including: — Name of the vaccine — Date of import or production — Expiration date — Production model number (Batch No.) — Average minimum-maximum temperature values and MKT values, which can be viewed in more detail at the lot level for each imported or produced batch. • The system must present the information daily, separating vaccine types for easy understanding and overview.
3. Distributor	• The system must display the number of all vaccines waiting to be shipped. • It should also display the minimum, maximum temperature, and MKT values as averages. • The system must provide information about vaccines waiting to be delivered, including the following: — Name of the distribution and transport company — Name of the vaccine waiting to be delivered — Number of vaccines waiting to be delivered, categorized by vaccine type — Date of receipt into the warehouse — Production model number (Batch No.)

(*Continued*)

Table 5.3. (*Continued*)

Functions and Operation of the System	Details
	— Minimum, maximum temperature values and MKT values, all presented as averages and can be drilled down to the vaccine type level. • The system must display the minimum, maximum temperature values, and daily MKT values (Warehouse Temperature by Date) in an easy-to-understand manner.
4. Delivery	• The system must display the total number of vaccines delivered. • It should also show minimum temperature and MKT values as averages. • Information on the number of vaccines delivered should be displayed, separated by the following: — Vaccine type — Production model number (Batch No.) • The system must also display the number of vaccines delivered: — Separated by the receiving hospital or medical facility • Detailed information on the number of vaccines delivered should include the following: — Name of the distribution and transport company — Name of the vaccine delivered — Number of vaccines delivered according to vaccine type — Delivery date — Production model number (Batch No.) — Minimum and maximum temperature values, as well as MKT values for each transport lot. • The system must present distribution information in a comprehensive and easily understandable way, separated by: — Vaccine type — Service area (Zone) — Province
5. Hospital	• The system must display information on the total number of vaccines waiting to be administered. • It should also show minimum, maximum, and MKT temperature values as averages.

Table 5.3. (*Continued*)

Functions and Operation of the System	Details
	• The system must display information on the number of vaccines waiting to be administered, divided by hospital. • The system must display information on minimum, maximum temperature, and MKT values, separated by hospital on a daily basis.
6. Vaccination	• The system must display information on the total number of vaccines administered, divided into first and second doses, as well as the total number of vaccination points. • The system must display information on the number of vaccines administered, separated by the following: — Date of injection — Hospital or injection point • The system must present this information in a comprehensive and easily understandable manner. The data should be separated by the following: — Type of person administering the injection (Person Type) — Gender — Service area (Zone) — Type of hospital (Hospital Type)
7. Serial	• The system must display detailed information about the vaccine, which includes the following: — Name of the vaccine — Production model number (Batch No) — Serial number — Date of import/production — Expiration date — Dates of various events, such as the import, storage in the company warehouse, and distribution to the hospital • Number of vaccines received by the hospital • Number of vaccines administered • Minimum and maximum temperature values and MKT values

(*Continued*)

Table 5.3. (*Continued*)

Functions and Operation of the System	Details
	• The system should also display injection information, which includes the following: — Production model number (Batch No) — Serial number — Injection date — Type of person administering the injection (Person Type) — Hospital or injection point — Injection needle (Dose nos. 1 and 2)

until January 2022, as announced by the government, in response to the COVID-19 virus epidemic, now considered an endemic disease (moving to COVID-19 endemic).

Government agencies have started utilizing vaccine traceability systems to enhance public safety. These systems can trace the distribution of vaccines, including their quantities and whether they have maintained a required temperature range. They are also capable of tracing problematic vaccines before their administration or distribution to patients. This not only reduces costs in logistics management but also lowers expenses resulting from the use of defective or poor-quality vaccines. Moreover, citizens can monitor the vaccine information they receive, fostering confidence in the vaccine's efficacy and quality through a platform system that monitors and traces the COVID-19 vaccine.

The research found that data standards and data sharing among relevant agencies (stakeholders) are crucial, along with their readiness to receive data. These are essential components for achieving effective tracking and traceability in the system. The system, an innovative full-cycle solution, can accurately track and trace vaccine information from upstream to downstream, linking with national agencies. It has been used in real-world scenarios to support decision-making and essential government policy formulation. This innovation differs from other domestic and foreign information technology systems related to traceability in the health industry. The research can serve as a development model and can be expanded to manage crises or emerging diseases.

5.2 Conclusion

This chapter showed that infrastructure is the backbone of hospital logistics, encompassing physical warehouses, transportation systems, and digital platforms. A particular focus was placed on cold chain logistics, which is essential for vaccines, blood, and other temperature-sensitive products. The COVID-19 pandemic served as a powerful case study, demonstrating how weaknesses in infrastructure can disrupt national health programs, while robust systems ensure that life-saving products are delivered intact.

The lesson from this chapter is that investment in infrastructure is not a luxury but a necessity. Reliable infrastructure improves service efficiency, reduces waste, and saves lives by protecting the integrity of sensitive products. Hospitals and healthcare systems must also build redundancy and flexibility into their logistics networks so they can adapt to emergencies such as pandemics or natural disasters. Ultimately, logistics infrastructure serves as a safeguard for both routine operations and crisis response.

Chapter 6

Cutting-Edge Research in Hospital Logistics

This chapter collects information on various aspects of hospital logistics research. The collected data from case study hospitals and research studies contribute to the application of logistics science in problem-solving. These studies have not only raised significant new issues but also explained newly discovered phenomena. They offer guidelines for problem-solving and various conclusions. These studies can serve as data models, and the concepts and results can be further developed in other hospitals.

6.1 CASE STUDY I: An Application of New Information Technology Systems in Hospital Logistics Systems (Kritchanchai *et al.*, 2018)

Currently, the hospital industry is expanding due to the increasing trend of an aging population (Kritchanchai *et al.*, 2018). This has led to heightened competition. Both private and public hospitals in Thailand are striving to improve their service delivery efficiency to seize opportunities in the medical service market. One of the strategies being employed is the application of new technology to various functions, notably to bolster the potential of the hospital's logistics system.

The goal of this research is to investigate how information technology systems are used in hospital supply chains. A qualitative survey was conducted across 20 community hospitals in Thailand. The study provides insights into the development of information technology systems in areas such as data management, data standardization, inventory management, the procurement process, and transportation management.

The research results indicated that hospitals with low efficiency often lack modern information technology systems in their logistics systems. Conversely, hospitals that effectively use information technology systems tend to have greater efficiency in their inventory management, procurement, and transportation processes.

6.1.1 *Basic information*

This study investigates the use of information technology systems in hospital supply chains, using data from a qualitative survey conducted in 20 Thai hospitals. The study particularly focuses on the role of these systems in the hospital product restocking process.

The research aims to answer the following questions:

(1) What benefits does the new information technology system offer in the hospital product replenishment process?
(2) Which kinds of organizations have the capacity to successfully deploy a new information technology system?

After examining 20 cases, we discovered that hospitals exhibit distinct characteristics in their use of information technology systems in fulfillment practices. We conducted the analysis with the assumption that information technology systems serve as the core of the product fulfillment process, which is linked to data standards, inventory, purchasing, and logistics processes. Effective data management can lead to improved efficiency in the product replenishment process.

6.1.2 *Study methods*

This qualitative survey collected data from 20 community hospitals, with bed sizes ranging from 60 to 200. The research aimed to gather in-depth information, leading to further inquiries. The survey questions targeted those responsible for or involved in product replenishment, purchasing, inventory, information technology, and transportation. Both individual interviews and direct observations were employed, using a structured format. The focus was on logistics activities within the hospital, including data management, data standardization, inventory management, purchasing processes, and transportation management. These elements relate to the replenishment process in the hospital supply chain, reflecting the use and capabilities of the information technology system in terms of inventory management, purchasing, and transportation processes.

6.1.3 *Study results*

This document is based on data collected from 20 hospitals. We conducted case studies by categorizing the information technology system capabilities of these hospitals' supply chain systems. A qualitative survey was conducted, allowing respondents to classify the steps involved in replenishing health service-supporting products. The questions were divided into five dimensions, each with four levels of answer criteria, as detailed below (Tables 6.1–6.5):

Table 6.1. Dimension 1 — this dimension pertains to the condition of data management.

Dimension 1: This dimension pertains to the condition of data management.	
Level 1	Utilizes a manual system for managing data flow and use standalone computer systems (i.e., computers that are not connected to other machines within the organization).
Level 2	Utilizes a computer system to manage the flow of information, but it remains an independent, separate system.
Level 3	Utilizes a computer system to manage the flow of information as an integrated system, but some connections are still manual.
Level 4	Utilizes the most modern information systems by using computers to manage the flow of information in an integrated manner, allowing data to be connected throughout the supply chain.

Table 6.2. Dimension 2 — This dimension involves establishing the level of data standardization.

Dimension 2: This dimension involves establishing the standardization level for data.	
Level 1	Defines standard codes used within the hospital, such as Product ID.
Level 2	Uses a method for matching other standard codes with internal hospital codes.
Level 3	Utilizes standard codes to link various codes in the hospital, like order codes, disbursement codes, and bar codes. Barcodes are applied in processes related to logistics.
Level 4	Applies the same standardized code using barcodes throughout the supply chain.

Table 6.3. Dimension 3 — This dimension relates to inventory management.

Dimension 3: This dimension is related to inventory management.	
Level 1	No forecasting system is used. Replenishment levels are based on preliminary estimates, and a manual system is utilized for recording data.
Level 2	A system is used to analyze and calculate replenishment levels. The data is recorded electronically but is stored in separate databases.
Level 3	Past data is analyzed in a systematic manner, and periodic adjustments are made to align with actual usage rates.
Level 4	Agencies responsible for storing specific products replenish those products in line with actual usage through Vendor Managed Inventory (VMI).

Table 6.4. Dimension 4 — This dimension relates to the status of purchasing.

Dimension 4: This dimension is related to the status of purchasing.	
Level 1	Fax, email, and/or telephone only.
Level 2	Fax, email, and/or telephone with a manual system for tracking product delivery situations.
Level 3	Use of the Electronic Data Interchange (EDI) system along with a manual system for tracking product delivery situations.
Level 4	An EDI system for communicating information and tracking the status of product orders with the product deliverer, covering the entire supply chain.

Table 6.5. Dimension 5 — This dimension relates to transportation management.

Dimension 5: This dimension relates to transportation management.	
Level 1	Utilize hospital employees (specifically, the department responsible for transportation) for goods transportation.
Level 2	Employ the central transportation agency for shipping and receiving goods within the hospital.
Level 3	Utilize the central transportation agency for shipping and receiving goods in the hospital, with the addition of tracking technology.
Level 4	Use the central transportation agency for shipping and receiving goods within the hospital. This level includes the use of tracking technology and continuous performance evaluation systems.

According to the interviews we conducted, those working in hospitals evaluate themselves based on certain competence levels. The results are shown in Table 6.6.

6.1.4 *Conclusion*

From the Table 6.6, we can see that most hospitals are at levels 1 and 2, some hospitals are at levels 2 and 3, but only a few hospitals are at levels 3 and 4. Therefore, we can group them into three groups as follows:

- Group 1 consists of two hospitals, Hospital No. 5 and Hospital No. 12, both operating at efficiency levels 3 and 4.
- Group 2 includes six hospitals, namely Hospitals 11, 14, 15, 16, 17, and 18, all operating at efficiency levels 2 and 3.
- Group 3 comprises 12 hospitals operating at performance levels 1 and 2. Based on this information, the following chart was generated.

In Group 1, we can observe the relationship between these five dimensions. When a hospital adopts standardized codes in its system, it is more likely to have an integrated information system across the institution. Since the entire supply chain has access to this information, forecasting systems are generally more effective. In a structured way, the hospital can use past data to calculate replenishment levels. However, no hospital in this group has yet implemented a vendor-managed inventory (VMI) system for the purchasing process. They

Table 6.6. Evaluation results of all 5 dimensions for 20 case study hospitals.

Dimension / Hospital	Data Management	Standardization Level	Inventory Management	Purchasing	Transportation Management
1	2	1	2	2	1
2	1	2	1	1	1
3	1	1	2	1	1
4	2	1	1	1	2
5	3	3	3	3	4
6	1	1	1	1	1
7	2	1	2	2	2
8	2	2	2	2	1
9	2	1	1	1	2
10	1	1	1	1	1
11	2	2	2	2	3
12	4	3	3	3	3
13	2	2	1	1	2
14	2	2	2	2	3
15	3	3	3	2	2
16	2	3	3	2	3
17	3	2	3	2	2
18	2	2	2	3	3
19	1	1	1	1	2
20	2	1	1	1	2

Notes: The score indicates the level of performance (the number 1 represents the lowest level and number 4 represents the highest level).

still rely on traditional, manual systems, but progress is evident. In this group, most hospitals have established a central transportation department to aid in managing internal transportation, resulting in improved efficiency.

Hospitals in groups 2 and 3 have implemented data standards and internal codes. However, their information management systems are often traditional and manual. As a result, the purchasing system is both traditional and manual. Data recording still relies on a manual system, using computers only to manage the flow of information and product replenishment. From my experience, the transportation management system is not very efficient. Most hospitals still depend on agencies for transportation as there is no established agency or logistics unit specifically responsible for this task.

The spider web diagrams depicted in Figures 6.1–6.4 illustrate the five-dimensional relationships among these 20 cases.

The results of all three groups indicate that the efficiency of **data standards** influences **data management systems**. When using internal codes, hospitals often have separate data systems, whereas when using data standards, linked information frequently occurs. This integration enables visibility of information throughout the supply chain. **Information management systems** also impact inventory **management and purchasing processes**. Computer systems and integration enhance forecasting system efficiency and lead to the application of Electronic Data Interchange (EDI). However, the absence of a dedicated logistics agency results in ineffective

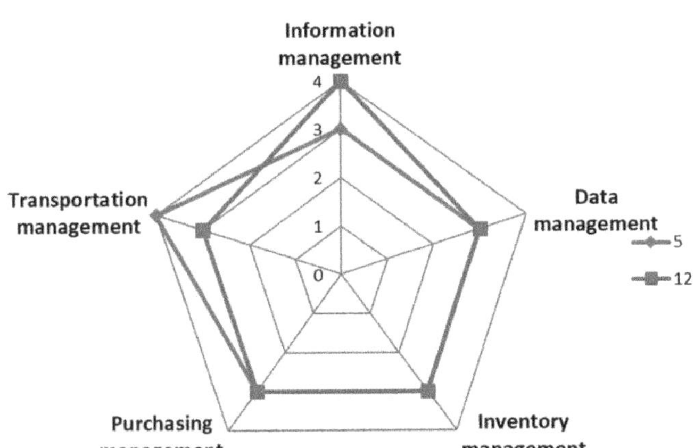

Figure 6.1. Group 1—Hospitals 5, 12.

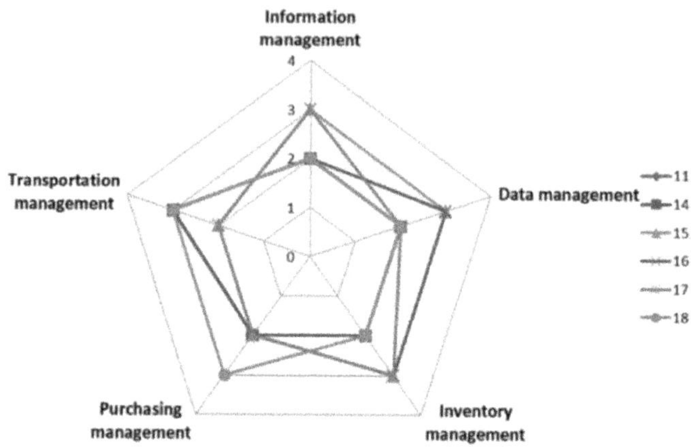

Figure 6.2. Group 2—Hospitals 11 and 14–18.

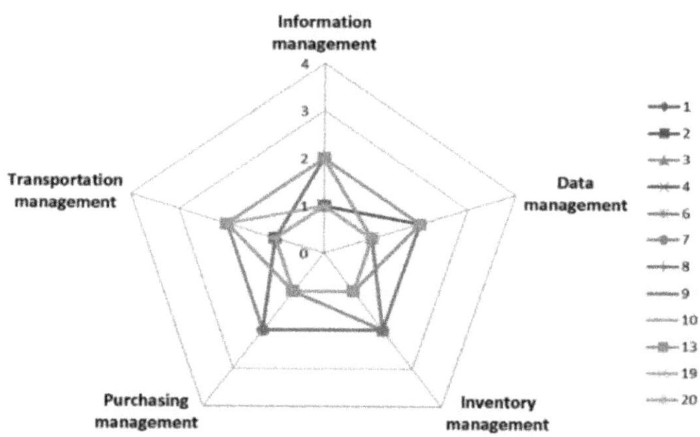

Figure 6.3. Group 3—Hospitals 1–4, 6–10, 13, and 19–20.

transportation management. Establishing a centralized transportation agency can improve intra-hospital transportation efficiency.

In response to the first research question about the benefits of the new information technology system, it was found that using this system, coupled with data standardization, forms the backbone of the product replenishment process. Effective use leads to efficient inventory management, purchasing, and transportation.

Regarding the second research question about the types of organizations that can successfully implement the new information technology system, surveys show that the strong performance of information

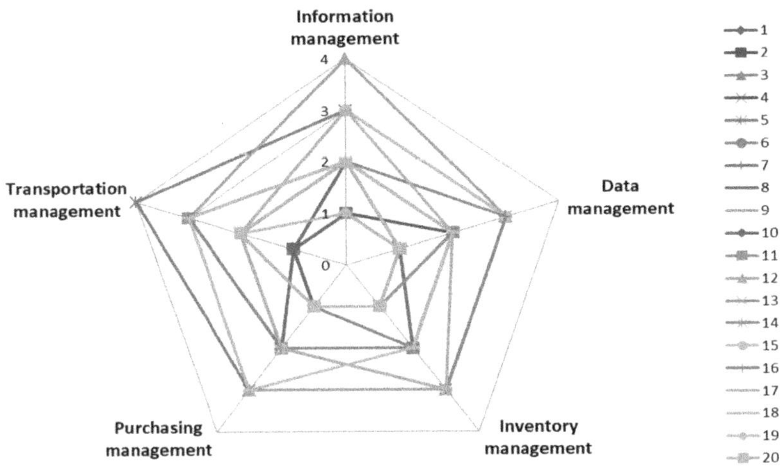

Figure 6.4. Evaluation results for five dimensions in 20 case study hospitals.

technology is not limited to high-quality computers or software systems. Instead, it hinges on data standards, which are fundamental for data linkage, integration, and visibility throughout the supply chain. Utilizing historical data for inventory management and improving the purchasing process's efficiency are made possible by these elements. The establishment of a central transport agency should be considered to achieve efficiency in the transportation system. The study reveals that the successful implementation of new information technology systems in Thai hospitals is also dependent on quality organizational processes.

6.2 CASE STUDY II: Creating a Simulation Model for the Allocation of Service Units in the Outpatient Department

This research develops the value chain concept, which breaks down activities in outpatient departments (OPDs) into primary and support activities. The study focuses on classifying OPD service units into main service units and support service units, demonstrating how to allocate these units based on the value chain concept.

When a new building was constructed, the research process began by observing patient flow in the outpatient department, which led to the relocation of some support service units. This change influenced the flow within the outpatient department. To study the effects of this change, the researchers employed the discrete-event simulation technique, examining activities in both the existing and new buildings.

The simulation results revealed that when a new building is constructed, and the main service units and support service units are separated, congestion in outpatient clinic areas can be relieved. Specifically, relocating the lab, X-ray, and drug dispensing units to the new building reduced congestion in the existing building area. Importantly, the simulation also indicated that the new building improved post-consultation processes by reducing waiting time and the number of waiting patients.

6.2.1 *Basic information*

The design of a new hospital building's service units significantly impacts its efficiency. The complexity of studying the design of these units inside the hospital building stems from the diverse activities and individuals involved. A well-designed service unit ensures adequate space for patient care and facilitates a smooth patient flow. Patient flow is a key factor in a health system that influences patient delays. Thus, an efficient patient flow is a significant indicator of hospital efficiency. Nonetheless, patient flow strongly correlates with service unit design due to the vast number of patients, distances to each location, and the variety of flows, routes, and destinations.

The primary goal of a patient's hospital visit is to receive treatment. This involves going through various service areas, such as registration, lab, finance, etc. Although the main purpose is to attend the clinic, other services cannot be eliminated from the process. This aligns with the concept of a value chain, where the main activities directly contribute to the final product or process result. Although support activities may not have a direct and substantial effect, they cannot be removed from the process.

This article combines patient flow behavior, service area allocation, and value chain models. The objective is to study the patient flow value chain, focusing on the main and supporting activities of the service units, along with the allocation of outpatient department service units in the newly constructed hospital building. Discrete simulation techniques are used to simulate patient flow from the moment they enter the hospital until they leave the outpatient department.

In a health system, the patient flow encompasses the entire patient journey, from arrival to departure. Incoming patients can either have appointments or walk-in without appointments. For instance, patients who wish to receive services from a clinic must receive diagnoses from various service points, including the lab. They then need to make payments at the finance office and collect their medications from the dispensary. Hence, according to the value chain concept, the main and supporting activities of service units allocated in the outpatient department can be classified as shown in Figure 6.5.

6.2.2 *Study methods*

6.2.2.1 *Development of flow concepts*

This study was conducted at a university hospital with 2,800 beds and 3,000,000 outpatients per year. The study focused on an outpatient department offering various services, including (1) primary, (2) orthopedic surgery, (3) general internal medicine, (4) obstetrics, (5) surgery, (6) preventive medicine, (7) dermatology, (8) ophthalmology, (9) ear,

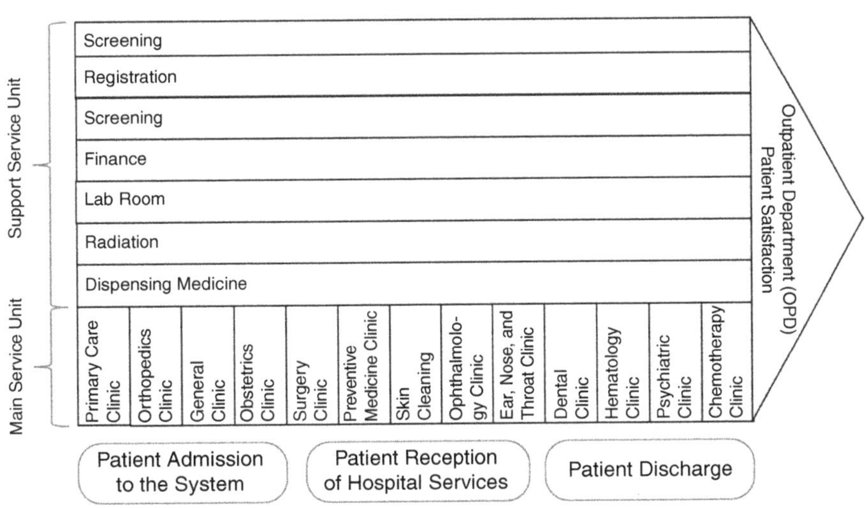

Figure 6.5. Outpatient flow value chain.

nose, and throat (ENT), (10) dentistry, (11) hematology, (12) psychiatry, and (13) a chemotherapy clinic. Additional service units include registration, screening, laboratory (Lab), X-ray room, medication, and payment units. Patients were classified into six groups:

1. Patients who did not make an appointment.
2. Patients undergoing lab work.
3. Patients having an X-ray.
4. Patients with an appointment who can walk unaided.
5. Patients with an appointment who use a wheelchair.
6. Patients waiting for appointments.

The flow of outpatients is illustrated in Figure 6.6.

6.2.2.2 *Model development*

The conceptual framework in Figure 6.6 served as the foundation for our research simulation. Yet, we modified the initial service units' allocation. All service units should be situated within one building, as Figure 6.7(a) illustrates. In the second scenario (Alternative), we dispersed the service units. As shown in Figure 6.7(b), we reassigned the support service unit, lab, X-ray, and drug dispensing unit to a new building.

The simulation's goal is to analyze congestion on each floor and plan service provision in alternative scenarios. The indicators include the following:

1. Each floor has a certain number of patients. We will separately calculate patient statistics in each category between the original situation and alternative scenarios.
2. The drug dispensing unit's number of patients, total duration, and utility in the new building. We will use this indicator to plan services in the new building.

6.2.2.3 *Inputting data into the model*

This research collected data by surveying the area and verifying numbers to use in simulating scenarios in the Arena program. The surveyed data include the number of patient arrivals (Figure 6.8), the service period for each activity, and the capacity of the services provided by the system.

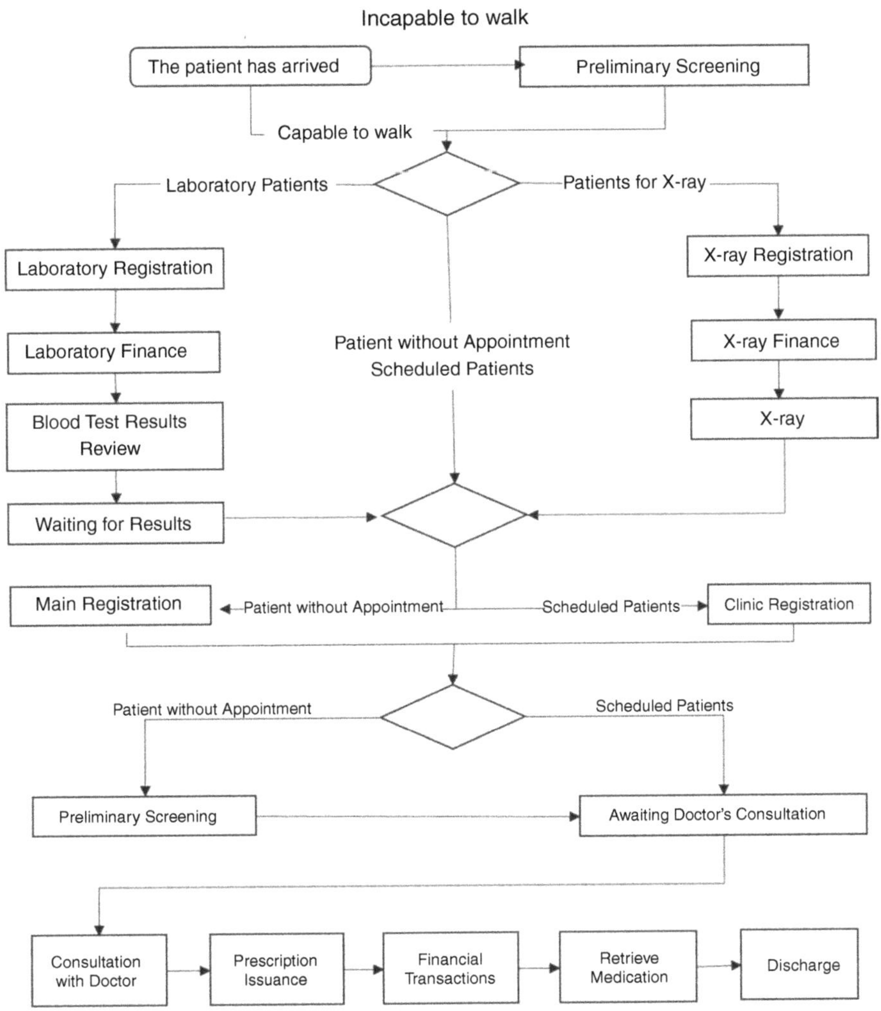

Figure 6.6. Conceptual framework for outpatient flow.

6.2.3 *Study results: Simulation results*

6.2.3.1 *Patient congestion*

We investigated patient crowding and the average length of time patients spend on each floor. A 2-sample t-test was used at a 5% significance level to test the following hypotheses:

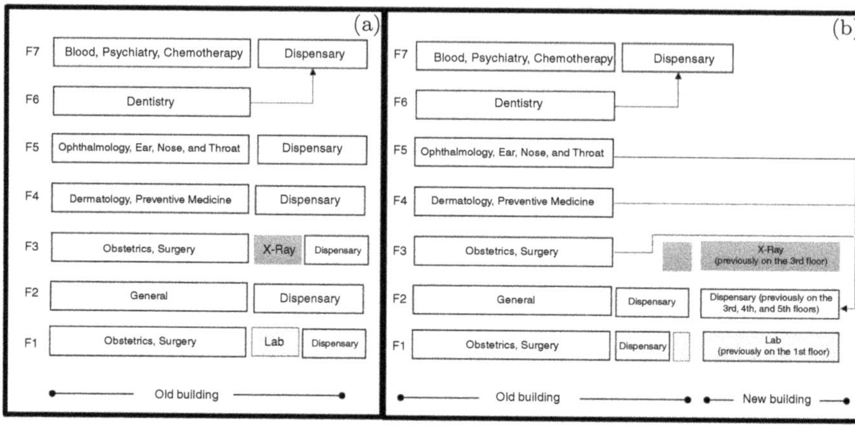

Figure 6.7. The original location of the service unit. (a) All service units should ideally be situated within the same building. (b) In alternative scenarios, service units may be separated.

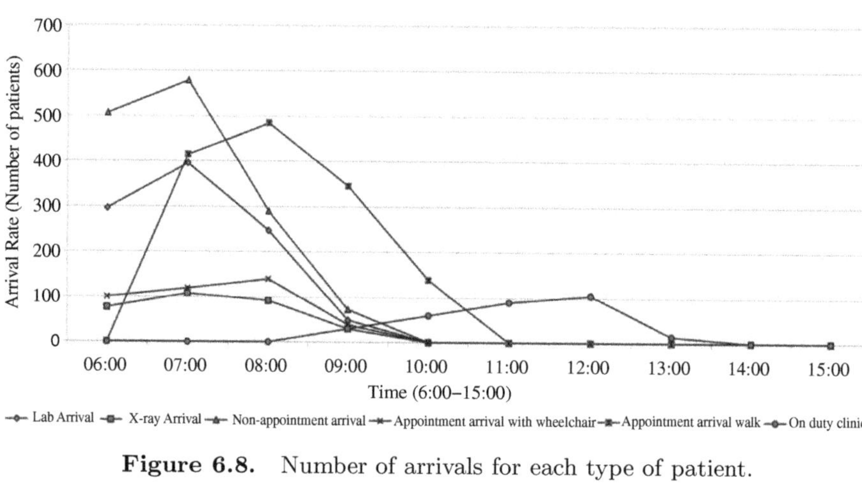

Figure 6.8. Number of arrivals for each type of patient.

— $\mathbf{H}_0$: The number of patients remains the same after separating the main service unit and the supporting service unit.

— $\mathbf{H}_1$: When the main service unit and the supporting service unit are separated, the number of patients changes.

The model's processing revealed that floors 1, 3, 4, and 5 rejected H_0. This implies that the separation of main service units and supporting service units statistically alters the patient count on these floors, resulting in a decrease in the number of patients.

6.2.3.2 *Resource allocation planning*

This study investigates how to plan the use of service units in new buildings. The model's processing found that despite improvements in Lab and X-ray checkpoints, patients still wait to see the doctor before undergoing tests. This is due to a bottleneck in the process of waiting to see a doctor. Ideally, the efficiency of doctors should be improved, but this is not feasible due to limitations in the case study hospital. Thus, we opted to consider improvements in the drug dispensing unit.

The drug dispensing unit is typically busy and operates with limited resources. To improve and develop the unit, it is necessary to increase the number of personnel, albeit modestly. Currently, an average of 319 patients wait approximately 104 minutes at the dispensary. To reduce total patient time, we suggest increasing the number of personnel in the unit to an optimal level. This level is defined as a dispensary service time not exceeding 30 minutes and a total number of waiting patients not exceeding 100.

The drug dispensing unit comprises a pharmacist, pharmacist assistant, and finance personnel, divided into two shifts as shown in Table 6.7.

The processing of the model reveals that the optimal allocation of resources for the morning hours (9:00–12:00) should include 3 pharmacist assistants, 3 financial officers, and 5 pharmacists to provide adequate services. The details are shown in Table 6.8.

Table 6.7. Allocation of work schedules and resources in the dispensary unit.

Period	Pharmacist Assistant	Financial Officer	Pharmacist
9:00–12:00	3	3	4
12:00–16:00	5	5	7

Table 6.8. Simulation model results for appropriate resource allocation scenarios.

Details	Optimum Value	Maximum Value
Total number of resources added	11 staff	48 staff
Total patient sessions in the dispensary unit	27.32 minutes	30 minutes
Total number of patients in the dispensary unit	85.68 staff	100 staff
Increase in the number of pharmacist assistants (9:00–12:00)	3 staff	8 staff
Increase in the number of pharmacist assistants (12:00–16:00)	0 staff	8 staff
Increase in the number of financial officers (9:00–12:00)	3 staff	8 staff
Increase in the number of financial officers (12:00–16:00)	0 staff	8 staff
Increase in the number of pharmacists (9:00–12:00)	5 staff	8 staff
Increase in the number of pharmacists (12:00–16:00)	0 staff	8 staff

6.2.4 *Conclusion*

This research aimed at two objectives. The first objective was to survey overcrowding among OPD patients under two conditions: (1) all service units must be in the same building and (2) we will classify service units into main and supporting units and allocate them to different buildings. The results indicated that moving support services (Lab, X-ray, and medicine dispensary unit) to a new building reduced congestion. There was a decrease in patients both before and after seeing a doctor, particularly on the 1st, 3rd, 4th, and 5th floors. On the first floor, congestion was reduced by relocating the room to the new building's first floor. Patients on the third floor experienced less congestion before seeing a doctor because fewer patients required X-rays.

Relocating the laboratory (Lab) and X-ray rooms proved beneficial, as these are usually the initial processes patients undergo before seeing a doctor. This moves reduced crowding among patients requiring lab and X-ray examinations and those waiting to see the doctor. On the 4th and 5th floors, patient congestion was reduced before clinic hours (9:00 a.m.) due to the separation of service units and the relocation of the drug dispensing unit to a new building. This allowed for better patient flow on 3rd, 4th, and 5th floors, reducing lengthy congestion.

The second objective was to plan an appropriate service allocation in the new building, with the goal of patients not needing to stay in the hospital after seeing a doctor. The service allocation in the existing and new buildings was determined based on the relocation of the lab, X-ray, and drug dispensing units to the new building. However, the services of the lab and X-ray room service unit remained unchanged. The most significant improvement was in the drug dispensing unit, which reduced the waiting time for drug dispensing to 27.32 minutes (from 104 minutes) and the number of patients on the drug dispensing floor at the new building to approximately 85.68 people (from 319 people). This was achieved by increasing the capacity with 3 pharmacist assistants (from the original 3), 3 financial officers (from the original 3), and 5 pharmacists (from the original 4) during the morning hours (9:00 a.m.–12:00 p.m.).

6.3 CASE STUDY III: Designing a Porter Management System within a Hospital

Managing stretcher shifts is a crucial logistical activity within hospitals. Many hospitals face challenges in this area, including an insufficient number of service providers and wheelchairs, leading to long waiting times for service recipients. Communication problems, such as repeated calls for service and busy phone lines, further exacerbate the issue. Additionally, there is often inadequate space for storing wheelchairs and insufficient personnel. The hub point's location for storing carts or serving as a central dispatch point also poses challenges. In response to these issues, a project was undertaken to improve and develop the stretcher shift management system within the hospital. The current shift management process was studied, and location analysis (hub location) was conducted. The resources, number of personnel, and amount of equipment suitable for the demand were analyzed. Recommendations were made for improving the business process of the on-call work group (patient movement), along with suggesting appropriate information technology (IT) solutions.

A hospital case study reveals that the patient transport service area simulation plan currently assigns seven service areas to the stretcher staff. The hospital has three stretcher service centers, referred to as HUBs, located in Building B, Building C, and Building D. Each stretcher service center, or HUB, is further divided into specific service areas or zones:

1. 1st Hub manages Building A and Building B's patient transport service areas.
2. 2nd Hub oversees the patient transport service areas of Building C, Building F, and Building G.
3. 3rd Hub is in charge of the patient transport service area of Building D and Building E.

Building H, a new building under construction, will be further analyzed for the possibility of establishing an additional HUB service center (Figure 6.9).

The staff and equipment at our facility consist of 37 individuals and various moving apparatuses, including 280 wheelchairs and 45 stretchers. These resources are distributed across three patient transfer centers, each with distinct operating hours:

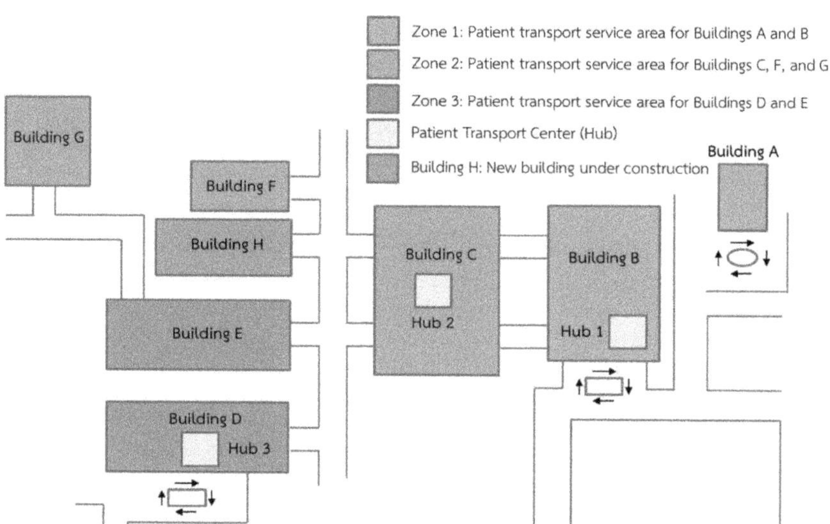

Figure 6.9. Patient transport service area simulation diagram (AS-IS).

— Patient Transfer Center 1st Hub operates in three shifts: 6:00 a.m.–8:00 a.m., 8:00 a.m.–4:00 p.m., and 4:00 p.m.–6:00 p.m.
— Patient Transport Center 2nd Hub operates during standard business hours, 8:00 a.m.–4:00 p.m.
— Patient Transfer Center 3rd Hub also has three shifts: 8:00 a.m.–4:00 p.m., 4:00 p.m.–12:00 a.m., and 12:00 a.m.–8:00 a.m.

The hospital's current workflow involves two channels for requesting stretcher services: 1st Channel at the outpatient building entrance (OPD) and 2nd Channel from various hospital departments. This process is manually managed. Work requests are accepted by filling out a patient referral form with the date, start time, patient's name and gender, transport equipment, destination, transporter number, and queue number. The transporter queue represents the daily work order, arranged on an A4 paper for staff reference. Once a transporter is assigned to a queue, they prepare the necessary equipment and travel to the patient's location. The patient is then delivered to their destination. Upon completion, the transporter returns to their service point and records their name and the time, thus concluding the process.

However, we have identified four key issues from staff brainstorming and Fish Bone Diagram analysis:

1. **Communication**: Multiple service requests lead to repeated calls, slow service, and busy phone lines.
2. **Staffing**: There are not enough staff members to meet service demands, especially during peak times.
3. **Evaluation**: There are no Key Performance Indicators (KPIs) to measure service provision.
4. **Equipment**: There are insufficient wheelchairs to meet patient demand, particularly during busy periods.

Addressing these issues requires comprehensive data analysis, including demand quantity, resource availability, shift center location, and business processes.

6.3.1 *Methods for analyzing patient transport center locations (hub)*

We can divide the methods for analyzing patient transport center locations into two scenarios.

Situation 1 involves finding a location for a patient transfer center (hub) by defining an operational zone of responsibility based on existing hospital policy (new hub/same zone).

Situation 2 involves finding both a location and a new operational zone of responsibility for the patient transport center (new hub/new zone). These techniques guide the analysis of patient transport center locations.

- **Situation 1**: Finding a new location (new hub/same zone)

We apply the mathematical model method to analyze the patient transport center location. This analysis is conducted using calculations in the Microsoft Excel program. We can conclude that Building B, Building C, and Building D should establish three patient transfer centers after processing the calculations in Microsoft Excel for situation 1. The goal is to minimize the product of distance and frequency of service calls, which results in the least overall patient movement. In creating the mathematical model, we specify indices (Indices), parameters (Parameters), and target equations (objective function) as follows:

Indices

i is a patient transfer center i ($i = 1, 2, 3$)
j is a building j ($j = 1, 2, 3, \ldots, 8$)

Parameters

S_{ij} is the distance from the patient transfer center i to the building j
D_{ij} is the frequency of service calls from the patient transfer center i to building j

Objective Function

$$\min_{\text{distance, demand}} \sum_i \sum_j S_{ij} D_{ij} X_{ij}. \qquad (1)$$

Equation (1) is the target equation for the patient transport center location, aiming to minimize the movement of patients from the patient transfer center i to building j.

- **Situation 2**: Finding a new location and zone (new hub/new zone)

We utilize the Center of Gravity Method to determine the location of the patient transfer center. This method helps us find a single location within a newly defined zone. The steps of this analysis are as follows:

1. We consider the appropriateness of service areas, which include the following:
   - Data on the quantity and frequency of patient transport center service calls
   - Information on distances between buildings
   - Work hours of the staff on duty
   - The special case of Building D, which must accommodate emergency patients
2. We set the latitude and longitude coordinates for each building.
3. We determine the frequency of service calls for each building.
4. Using a specific calculation formula, we determine the location of the patient transport center.

$$\text{Coordinates } X = \frac{\sum_{j=1}^{n} X_j D_j}{\sum_{j=1}^{n} D_j}, \tag{2}$$

$$\text{Coordinates } Y = \frac{\sum_{j=1}^{n} Y_j D_j}{\sum_{j=1}^{n} D_j}, \tag{3}$$

where

X_j is the latitude coordinates of building j,
Y_j is the longitude coordinates of building j,
D_j is the frequency of service calls for building j,
n is the number of buildings.

6.3.2 *Method for analyzing resource allocation within a patient transport center*

The analysis of resource allocation within the patient transport center can be divided into three scenarios: worst-case, base-case, and best-case. Each scenario can be further divided according to the type of resource: wheelchairs, stretchers, and staff. The calculation steps for all patient transport centers are as follows:

1. Determine the average resource service time for one cycle, based on area surveys and interviews with staff. For instance, allocate 120, 150, and 180 minutes for wheelchairs and stretchers, and allocate 8, 10, and 15 minutes for staff shifts.
2. Calculate the number of cycles needed to service the resource. This is done by dividing the work time into one-hour increments (60 minutes) by the average resource service time per cycle. For instance, in a period of one hour (60 minutes), resources can be provided half a time (0.5 times).

   The number of rounds needed to provide resources is

   $$\frac{60}{120} = 0.5 \text{ rounds}$$

3. Choose the resource service frequency:
   - The worst-case scenario selects the highest resource service frequency (maximum demand).
   - The base-case scenario chooses the average daily resource service frequency (average demand).
   - The best-case scenario picks the least resource service frequency (minimum demand).
4. Calculate the appropriate number of resources for each work period. This is done by dividing the frequency of resource service in each period by the number of cycles needed to service the resource obtained from step 2.
5. Select the number of resources in the time period that calculates the largest number of resources.

6.3.3 *Calculation results: Location of patient transport center*

The analysis results were divided into three scenarios.

- Scenario 1: Find a new hub while using the same service area or zone (4 Hubs).
- Scenario 2: Find a new hub while using the same area or service zone (3 Hubs).
- Scenario 3: Choose a new hub with a new service area or zone.

From the analysis, it was concluded that the hospital should consider Scenario 2. This is because the demand for patient transport

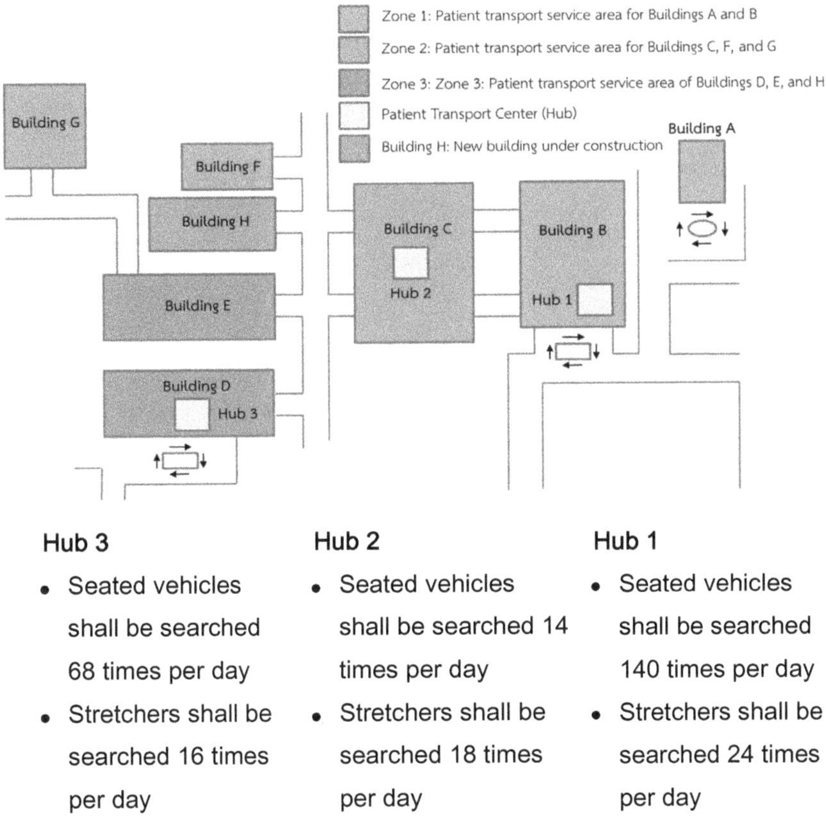

Figure 6.10. Patient transport service area simulation diagram proposed.
Source: LogHealth, Mahidol University. (2022). Design of Logistics Management and Services System at Somdejprapinklao Hospital, Royal Thai Navy (Porter management system and Inventory Management Information System) Project.

center services in each operational zone is similar. The location of the patient transport center in Scenario 2 is depicted in Figure 6.10.

We will apply the mathematical model method to analyze the location of the patient transfer center. This is divided into three service zones:

- Zone 1 includes Building A and Building B.
- Zone 2 consists of Building C, Building F, and Building G.
- Zone 3 encompasses Building D, Building E, and Building H. Building H is designated Zone 3 due to its high service call frequency from Buildings D and E. This is based on a comparison

Table 6.9. Results of the location of the patient transport center (Hub) from Microsoft Excel.

To \ From	Demand × Distance		
	Building B	Building C	Building D
Building A	80,513.16	70,932.61	1,15,561.04
Building B	21,941.24	17,323.60	62,549.90
Building C	26,017.60	14,230.10	45,419.50
Building D	95,218.76	45,931.75	13,121.78
Building E	47,429.60	14,257.00	31,321.50
Building F	70,974.72	29,934.32	50,430.94
Building G	1,23,498.76	64,907.01	72,979.76
Building H	56,992.28	20,624.23	41,224.68

of the number of Building H's estimated beds with data on the quantity and frequency of service calls from Buildings D and E.

The analysis of patient transport center locations uses data on the quantity and frequency of service calls (demand) and distance details (distance). The goal is to have the lowest value when multiplying the distance by the frequency of service calls, resulting in the least overall patient movement.

We can conclude that Building B, Building C, and Building D should establish three patient transfer centers after processing the calculations for situation 2 (Table 6.9).

The location analysis for scenario 2 (new hub/old zone—3 hubs) of the patient transport center provides the following insights:

— **Patient Transport Center at Building B (Hub 1):** Handles service areas in Building A and Building B.
— **Patient Transfer Center at Building C (Hub 2):** Takes care of service areas in Buildings C, F, and G.
— **Patient Transport Center at Building D (Hub 3):** Manages service areas in Buildings D and E.

By comparing the patient transfer service area simulation plans before and after the analysis of the patient transfer center location for Scenario 2, it is clear that while the location of the patient transfer center remains the same, the service area under its responsibility increases at Building D (Hub 3), also known as Building H.

Table 6.10. The count of wheelchairs and stretchers, as identified from the analysis for each patient transport center in the baseline scenario, within a span of a 120 minutes period.

Hub	Type	No. of Resource	
		AS-IS	Proposed
Building B	Wheelchair	222	140
	Hospital bed	43	24
Building C	Wheelchair	5	14
	Hospital bed	3	18
Building D	Wheelchair	3	68
	Hospital bed	1	16
Total	Wheelchair	230	222
	Hospital bed	47	58

6.3.4 *Results of resource calculation for the patient transfer center*

- **Resources for wheelchairs and stretchers:** The analysis suggests that hospitals should prepare wheelchairs and stretchers based on the base-case scenario. This is under the assumption that one round trip takes 120 minutes, which is the average usage time for these vehicles. This information comes from a survey of the area and interviews with stretcher personnel, as shown in Table 6.10.

From Table 6.10, we can conclude the following:

— **Patient Transport Center at Building B (Hub 1)**: The hospital needs to prepare for 140 wheelchairs and 24 stretchers per day.
— **Patient Transport Center at Building C (Hub 2)**: The hospital needs to prepare for 14 wheelchairs and 18 stretchers per day.
— **Patient Transport Center at Building D (Hub 3)**: The hospital needs to prepare for 68 wheelchairs and 16 stretchers per day.

In total, the hospital needs to prepare for 222 wheelchairs and 58 stretchers per day. This is **close to** the number of resources currently available, requiring the addition of 11 stretchers. Based on these results, the hospital must also consider how to allocate resources at each transport center.

- **Resources related to personnel:** Based on the calculation results, hospitals should prepare their staff according to the base-case scenario, assuming that one round trip takes an average of 10 minutes. This is the typical duration for staff to serve patients, as indicated by patient transport slips and interviews with stretcher shift staff. The data can be found in Table 6.11.

Based on Table 6.11, the following staffing requirements are suggested:

1. **Patient Transport Center at Building B (Hub 1):** The hospital should consider the following staff allocation.
   a. From 6:00 a.m. to 8:00 a.m., assign 3 operating staff.
   b. From 8:00 a.m. to 4:00 p.m., assign 4 operating staff.
   c. From 4:00 p.m. to 6:00 p.m., assign 1 operating staff.
2. **Patient Transport Center at Building C (Hub 2):** The hospital should consider the following staff allocation.
   a. From 8:00 a.m. to 4:00 p.m., assign 5 operating staff.

Table 6.11. Number of staff derived from the analysis (people) for each patient transport center (Base-Case) in Scenario 2 (with a service time of under 10 minutes).

Hub	Shift (Period Time)	No. of Resource	
		AS-IS	Proposed
Building B (Hub 1)	6.00-8.00	8	3
	8.00-16.00	18	4
	16.00-18.00	3	1
Building C (Hub 2)	8.00-16.00	6	5
Building D (Hub 3)	8.00-16.00	3	7
	16.00-18.00	1	1
	0.00-8.00	1	1

3. **Patient Transfer Center at Building D (Hub 3):** The hospital should consider the following staff allocation.
   a. From 8:00 a.m. to 4:00 p.m., assign 7 operating staff.
   b. From 4:00 p.m. to 12:00 a.m., assign 1 operating staff.
   c. From 12:00 a.m. to 8:00 a.m., assign 1 operating staff.

In conclusion, the hospital should allocate 18 operating staff per day, which is less than the current number available. This suggests that the current staffing levels are sufficient to meet demand.

6.3.5 *New format business process design results (business process)*

The business process design for patient transport work employs IT systems to enhance management and efficiency. The platform development comprises three parts: Part 1 is a web application for moving centers; Part 2 is a mobile application for shift workers; and Part 3 is a web application for various agencies (Figure 6.11).

The new business process format begins with service calls originating from two sources. The first source is the Patient Transfer

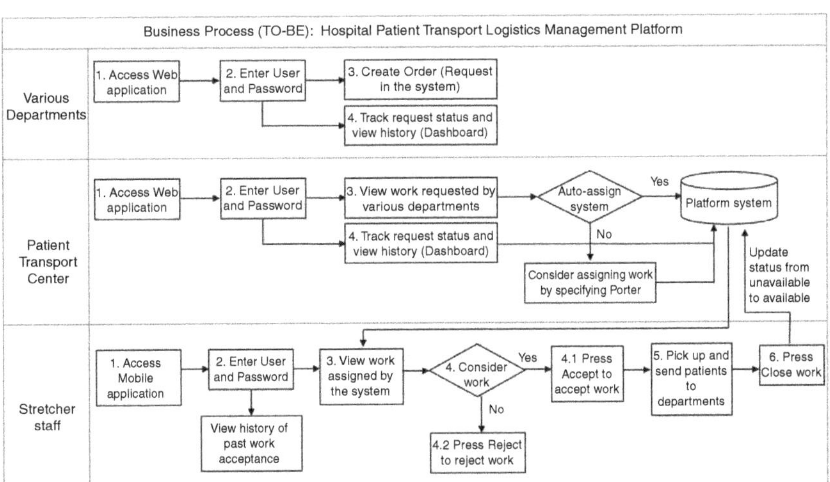

Figure 6.11. Proposed business process.
Source: LogHealth, Mahidol University. (2022). Design of Logistics Management and Services System at Somdejprapinklao Hospital, Royal Thai Navy (Porter management system and Inventory Management Information System) Project.

Center (Hub). When patients access the service, staff at each center create service requests via a web application. The second source includes various departments that also create service requests through the web application to arrange patient pickups. Once the system receives a service request, an administrator from each patient transport center assigns work tasks based on the service area. There are two types of work assignment formats:

1. **Automatic work assignment:** The system sends the task to the stretcher worker closest to the patient's location. It considers the worker's past assignments.
2. **Custom work assignments:** The center staff (Admin) can specify which shift worker should pick up the order.

Shift workers receive job orders via a mobile application. They can choose to accept or reject the assignment. If rejected, the system will assign the task to another worker. If approved, the stretcher worker prepares to move the patient. After successfully delivering the patient to their destination, the stretcher worker marks the job as completed in the mobile application, changing their status from unavailable to free. Various departments can then rate the service after the job is closed. All information is stored on the platform. Different departments can track work status and service call history via the dashboard.

6.3.6 *Results of software function design*

When designing information technology systems, the functions of the software should include those listed in Table 6.12:

6.3.7 *Dashboard design results*

By studying software systems composed of various components, you can understand the key features and details of software functions. This knowledge can be used to design a display screen or dashboard, as depicted in Figures 6.12 and 6.13.

- **Job Status Snapshot**
  - Number of jobs created at the defined time
  - Number of ongoing jobs at the defined time

Table 6.12. Details of software functions.

Task Overview	Detailed Description	Remark
Software Functionalities		
Web application for Managing Patient Movement	— Comprehensive data on each patient transfer center — Department-specific information — Profiles of patient transfer center staff — User rights and access parameters — Stretcher staff history — Record of previous service interactions — Interactive dashboard — Criteria for receiving and dispatching services — Service step management — Service request feature — Automated work distribution to stretcher staff — Custom work allocation to stretcher staff — Real-time tracking of progress — Service quality evaluation — Data gathering and visualization of service history	Compatibility with Google Chrome
Mobile application for Stretcher Staff	— Identity registration and verification — Personal history data settings — Work status of stretcher staff — Accepting work assignments — Concluding work assignments — Declining work assignments — Management of service steps — Record of past service and performance rating	Compatibility with iOS and Android
Web application for Various Departments	— Department Assignment — Service delivery terms — Service process management — Service request feature — Service quality evaluation — Record of service usage	Compatibility with Google Chrome

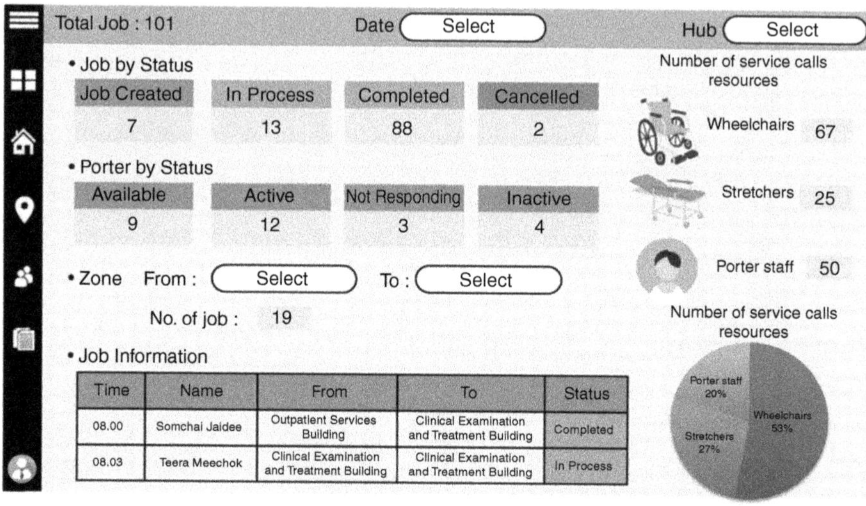

Figure 6.12. Example of a wheelchairs/stretchers/officer dashboard.

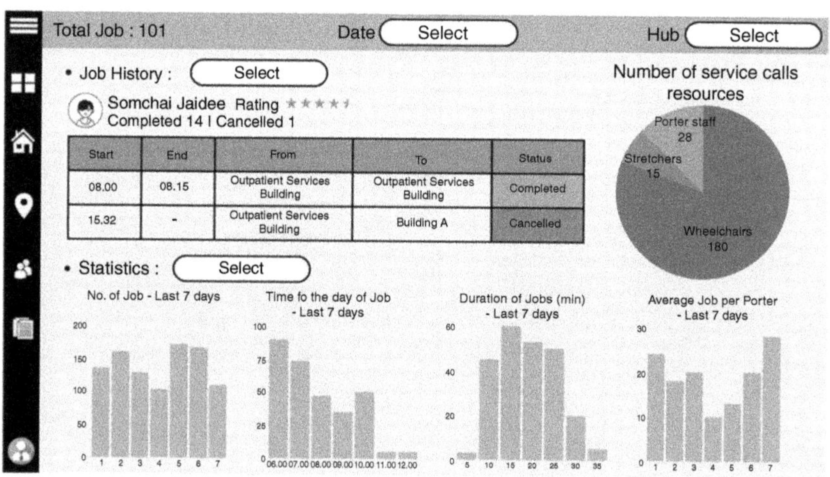

Figure 6.13. Statistics on historical usage of wheelchairs, stretchers, and staff dashboard.

Source: Log Health, Mahidol University. (2022). Design of Logistics Management and Services System at Somdejprapinklao Hospital, Royal Thai Navy (Porter management system and Inventory Management Information System) Project.

  - Number of completed jobs at the defined time
  - Number of canceled jobs at the defined time

- **Porter Status Snapshot**
  - Number of available stretcher officers
  - Number of staff currently engaged in duties
  - Number of stretcher officers not responding
  - Number of idle stretcher staff

- **Zone Area Selection**
  - Enables selection of starting and ending areas for potential work volume display

- **Job Details**
  - Provides full details about the job
  - Service duration
  - Officer on duty
  - Starting point
  - Destination
  - Status: Current job status (created, in progress, completed, and canceled)

- **Resource Service Call Count**. This shows the number of resource service calls, divided into categories:
  - Wheelchairs Category
  - Stretchers Category
  - Staff Category

- **Proportion of Resource Service Calls**. This represents the ratio of resource service calls, divided into the following categories:
  - Wheelchairs Category
  - Stretchers Category
  - Staff Category
  - Category

- **Number of Resources Available:** Displays the number of available resources, categorized by type, such as wheelchairs, stretchers, or porters. This is displayed according to the selected hub.

- **Job History (when Selecting a Stretcher Staff):** Provides an overview of the stretcher staff's history, including the following.
  - Rating: Points received for providing services
  - Total completed service workload
  - Total rejected workload
  - Service start time
  - Service end time
  - Origin
  - Destination
  - Work status (executed/canceled)
- **Statistics:** Allows you to select a period to display past service call results, such as the last 7 days, last week, or last month. This includes the following, as shown in Figure 6.13:
  - Job Count — Last 7 days: Shows the total number of jobs called for service in the past 7 days.
  - Job Time of Day — Last 7 days: Shows the number of jobs called for service, segmented by time of day, in the past 7 days.
  - Job Duration (min) — Last 7 days: Shows the number of jobs called for service in the past 7 days, categorized by duration.
  - Average Job Per Porter — Last 7 days: Shows the average workload for porters over the past 7 days.

6.4 Conclusion

Hospital logistics is evolving rapidly thanks to research and innovation. This chapter introduced technologies such as simulation modeling, time-driven activity-based costing, digital twins, and artificial intelligence as tools to enhance efficiency and planning accuracy. Research findings revealed how these approaches can reduce costs and improve service delivery, especially in high-demand areas such as outpatient departments.

The key lesson from this chapter is that while technology offers immense potential, its success depends on integration with hospital processes and staff readiness. Innovations cannot simply be copied from industry. They must be tailored to the healthcare environment, where patient safety and regulatory compliance are paramount. Evidence-based approaches, supported by pilot projects and careful evaluation, ensure that new systems deliver real benefits. Research and innovation, therefore, serve as catalysts for hospitals to adapt to future challenges.

Chapter 7

Best Practices in Hospital Logistics Systems

This chapter examines logistics systems in model hospitals. The examples originate from the "Train the Trainer: Logistics in Hospital" curriculum project. This project aims to educate and develop hospital personnel in logistics, enabling them to apply this knowledge to problem-solving and improve hospital logistics processes. In addition, these trained individuals act as representatives, transferring logistics knowledge to other personnel within the hospital. Implementation of this project can bring about change within the hospital, leading to enhanced efficiency. It helps reduce inventory value, which results in more efficient financial management. It also lessens service recipient waiting time, eliminates unnecessary steps in the supply chain (for medicine, medical supplies, and other items), and decreases product waiting time (lead time). The application of the ABC analysis technique can reduce the amount of new medicine and medical supply reserves. The project also focuses on developing transportation processes within hospitals to utilize human resources and transportation equipment in the most efficient manner. We discuss these processes in detail for all 16 hospitals as follows (Table 7.1):

Table 7.1. Survey data of 16 hospitals.

Model	Number of Beds	Logistics Project		
		Development of Inventory Management System	Development of a Central Transportation Agency and Increasing the Efficiency of the Transportation System	Improving the Efficiency of the Patient Transport System and Reducing Outpatient Waiting Times
1. Hospital A	150	✓		
2. Hospital B community	60	✓		
3. Hospital C	528	✓		
4. Hospital D community	89	✓		
5. Hospital E	121	✓		
6. Hospital F	850	✓	✓	
7. Hospital G community	38	✓		
8. Hospital H	700	✓		
9. Hospital I community	60	✓		
10. Hospital J	924			✓
11. Hospital K	600	✓	✓	
12. Hospital L community	80	✓	✓	
13. Hospital M	600	✓	✓	
14. Hospital N	252	✓	✓	
15. Hospital O	601	✓	✓	
16. Hospital P	875		✓	

7.1 Results of the Study of Prototypes for Developing Logistics Systems in Hospitals

A. Hospital A (Hospital size: 150 beds)

Hospital D, located in Suphanburi Province, is a level M2 (Middle-level) network community hospital with a capacity of 150 beds. It provides health services to the public in the U-Thong District and nearby areas. It also offers continuous care in all four main medical

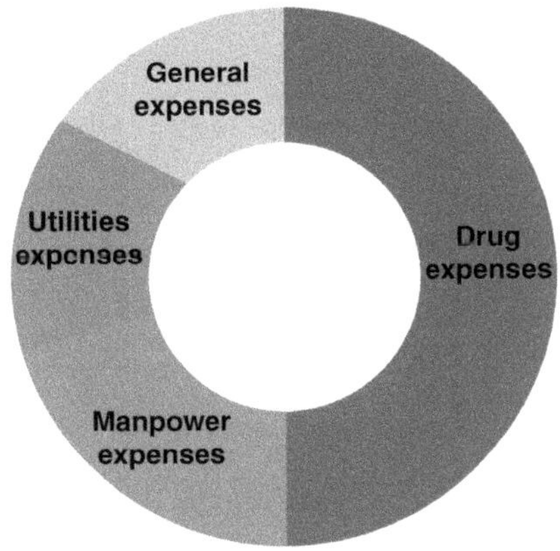

Figure 7.1. Hospital expenses A.
Source: Adapted from Hospital logistics management, by D. Kritchanchai and S. Srisakunwan, 2023, Healthcare Supply Chain Excellence Centre (LogHealth), Mahidol University.

fields. The hospital has a network of 22 subdistrict health promotion hospitals. It employs a total of 468 people, including 18 full-time doctors, 7 dentists, 15 pharmacists, and 118 professional nurses, among others (data from 2012–2015).

❖ From late 2015, the hospital has been in a level-7 financial crisis (the most severe level) for two consecutive quarters. The principal expenses include general costs, utilities, labor, and medication, which comprise the highest expenses category (Figure 7.1).

A.1 *Project: Improving the efficiency of drug warehouse management*

A.1.1 *Basic information and problem conditions*

The hospital has undergone a level-7 financial crisis (the most severe level) for two consecutive quarters according to official financial reports. The major expenses include general living expenses, utilities, manpower, and medication costs. The latter is the highest expense. The problems related to drug warehouse management are as follows:

- Counting stock is a time-consuming process.
- Information on the quantity of medicines in the warehouse is imprecise and unreliable.

- Current reserve estimates are inadequate. Overstocking of certain medicines and medical supplies has resulted in some products deteriorating or expiring.
- Some subdivisions have withdrawn more than the necessary amount.
- The front-of-house (Front Office) and back-of-house (Back Office) information systems are not interconnected.

A.1.2 *Improvement strategies (Figure 7.2)*

1. To manage inventory more efficiently, the hospital has developed an information system known as the Hospital Enterprise Resource Planning (ERP) program. This program, designed and developed in-house, serves as a data link. It collects information and creates a database, mapping the database of drug and medical supply warehouses (Drug 5.4 program). Furthermore, it links data at drug dispensing points (the HosXp program).
2. Design new work processes in line with the hospital ERP program for emerging needs:

    - To calculate the quantity of drugs and medical supplies needed from the warehouse, the program will do the calculations that previously required manual calculations by staff.
    - Recording on the medication withdrawal form can be done by printing it from the program. This replaces the old process where officials had to record the information manually and personally deliver it to the drug warehouse.
    - In terms of drug transportation, the warehouse staff responsible for refilling medicines in various departments, including the outpatient and inpatient medicine rooms, will use the program. Previously, this task required coordination between different medicine rooms and manual tracking of medicines and supplies for each withdrawal.

A.1.3 *Operation results*

(1) Information systems at the front (front office) and back (back office) of the house are linked. This allows the drug warehouse to monitor the status and remaining quantities of medicines in the outpatient (OPD) and inpatient (IPD) medicine rooms.

(2) The counting and disbursement process in the (OPD) and (IPD) medicine rooms is quicker. (Originally taking 1–2 days, it now takes only 30 minutes.)
(3) The value of inventory in the large medicine warehouse, (OPD), and (IPD) medicine rooms has been reduced. (The overall amount decreased from 9 million baht to 6 million baht.)
(4) Inventory counting is faster and more accurate.
(5) Drug shortages, excess stock, and expired drugs have all been reduced.
(6) The financial crisis level has been reduced from 7 to 3, improving the hospital's financial position.

B. Hospital B (community hospital with 60 beds)

Hospital B is a medium-sized community hospital situated in Ratchaburi Province, on the border with Myanmar. It falls under the Level F-2 classification and can accommodate up to 60 patients. At present, there are no specialized doctors, and there is a rotation of medical staff every two years. The hospital employs a total of 198 people, including 7 doctors, 8 dentists, 4 pharmacists, and 50 professional nurses, among others. It serves a population of 59,736 people in its coverage area (data from 2015).

B.1 *Project: Reducing the cost of drug and medical supplies inventory*

B.1.1 *Basic information and problem conditions*

1. The inventory reserve exceeds the required amount, resulting in a loss of opportunity for fund circulation and increased storage costs. This has caused a level-1 financial crisis in the hospital. Despite maintaining a 1.5-month supply of products to cater to service recipients and account for seller delivery variations, there are instances of product shortages and returns. Some products have also deteriorated or expired.
2. The purchasing process is plagued by issues such as lengthy procurement times due to late product delivery from sellers, incorrect deliveries as per the purchase order, and product shortages. The internal approval process from the director also presents challenges.

3. In the drug disbursement process, a concrete plan is yet to be established. Currently, there is only a set maximum quantity for each product type. For instance, the disbursement cycle is fixed for two weeks, and the maximum quantity stored is enough for two weeks of usage. However, there are occasions where the supply is insufficient, forcing service units to borrow goods from nearby units.

B.1.2 *Improvement strategies*

1. Refine the purchasing process to minimize lead time.
   1.1 Utilize value stream mapping to assess logistics processes, identify issues, and implement business process reengineering in the purchasing process. This includes identifying needs and issuing purchase orders, as well as approvals and inspections.
   1.2 Decrease purchasing processing time to reduce product lead time.
2. Utilize the ABC analysis technique to establish the quantity of new drug and medical supply reserves.
   2.1 The hospital employs the ABC analysis technique to categorize products based on their importance, taking into account their warehouse value. This technique aids in determining an appropriate quantity of product reserves, allowing for an understanding of product quantities by hospital group. Aim to reduce the Group A products' reserve from 1.5 months to one month.
3. Implement Kanban techniques to help with stock counting and efficient product replenishment.
   3.1 Hospitals apply Kanban, a technique in the Just-in-Time product management system, by attaching Kanban cards to products. For instance, attaching one Kanban card to 10 products enhances the efficiency of stock counting. This technique reduces stock counting time and promotes efficient product replenishment.
4. Change the frequency of disbursements from every two weeks to once a week.

B.1.3 *Operation results*

1. The value of inventories, including drugs and medical supplies, decreased by 20%.

2. Products such as medications and medical supplies are in short supply.

C. Hospital C (528 beds)

Hospital C, located in Bangkok, is a government hospital under the Department of Medical Services, Ministry of Public Health. It provides tertiary-level or higher medical services and has 600 beds across 28 wards. On average, the hospital provides 51,000 outpatient and 2,150 inpatient services per month. Currently, the hospital staff, including medical and other personnel, totals 1,700 people. This includes 114 doctors, 12 dentists, 548 professional nurses, 45 pharmacists, and other staff (2017 data).

C.1 *Project: Develop a material inventory management system for medical materials*

C.1.1 *Basic information and problem conditions*

1. There are concerns about shortages and surpluses of medical materials in stock. This is because the level of demand varies depending on the service recipient and changes over time.
2. There is a mismatch between the information in the warehouse management system and the actual quantity of parcels in the warehouse. This results in the incomplete delivery of medical materials to wards or service units due to a lack of proper stock verification.

C.1.2 *Improvement strategies*

1. The hospital has standardized the material balance and duplicate codes to ensure consistency between the hospital program system and the warehouse. This is achieved by using the same unit of measurement across all departments.
2. Adjustments have been made to the business process for disbursing medical supplies to make it more appropriate.
3. A system has been established to control the inventory of medical supplies. This includes establishing a maximum stock level to prevent excessive storage, as well as defining a new reorder point and safety stock level. This ensures that there are sufficient medical supplies available without causing a shortage.

C.1.3 *Operation results*

1. The material unit system uses the smallest units uniformly across the board.
2. The information about medical materials in the warehouse system and the supplies account is accurate and consistent.
3. The quantity of stored medical supplies has decreased.
4. Workers' satisfaction with withdrawing medical materials has improved, as the procurement department has sufficient medical materials on the pilot list to meet demand from multiple agencies.
5. The use of paper has been reduced, decreasing the workload associated with patient care activities related to withdrawing and receiving materials.
6. The expenses for purchasing medical supplies have been reduced by 2.7 million baht.
7. The cost of expired products has been reduced by 230,000 baht. This has resulted in accurate, reliable, and verifiable information, as well as increased storage space because of sufficient supplies.

D. Hospital D (community hospital with 89 beds)

Located in Chiang Dao District, Chiang Mai Province, Hospital D serves as a community hospital. With 89 beds, it provides care and services to a total of 103,790 people in the area. The staff includes 10 doctors and 58 professional nurses, based on 2016 data.

D.1 *Project: Develop a system for stockpiling and distributing drugs in hospitals*

D.1.1 *Basic information and problem conditions*

1. The hospital has observed that the subdispensing unit is withdrawing drugs based on experience and prediction, leading to two primary problems. This can sometimes result in larger doses being withdrawn than necessary, creating a product hoarding situation. Other times, there is a shortage of medicine to fulfill the needs, causing an imbalance between the amount of medicine needed and the amount in reserve. The subdrug warehouse often withdraws additional drugs outside of the specified timeframe, leading to an increased workload for the drug warehouse staff, as medicine must be distributed on multiple trips.

2. There are issues with the current information system. In the hospital's drug management, there are two systems: the Drug program, used for the main drug warehouses, and the HOSxP system, used for drug storage and dispensing medicine to patients. These two systems do not share information. As a result, when medicines are disbursed to the subdrug warehouses, including the outside, inside, and Non-Communicable Diseases (NCDs) medicine rooms, the main drug warehouse cannot inspect the system. They determine the actual balance and usage rate of the various drug warehouses, which affects purchasing planning and inventory management. Additionally, there are instances when drugs are withdrawn from a smaller drug warehouse without recording the information. This prevents the actual usage rate from being known, affecting drug reserves in both large and small drug warehouses and leading to imbalances.

D.1.2 *Improvement strategies (Figure 7.2)*

1. Modify the large medicine warehouse's medication withdrawal schedule. Previously, withdrawals occurred every four weeks, leading to excessive stockpiling at the drug depot. Now, withdrawals take place weekly from three service points: the external medicine room, the internal medicine room, and the NCDs medicine room, all of which are located directly from the large medicine warehouse.

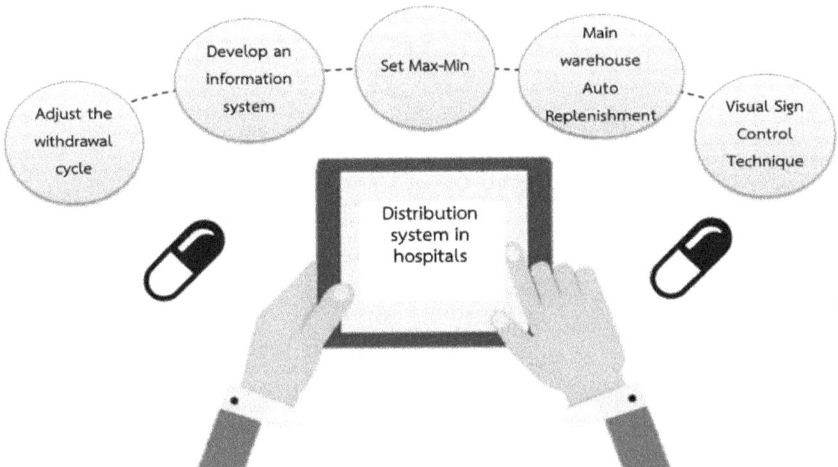

Figure 7.2. Improvement strategies for the hospital drug distribution system.

2. Implement an information system capable of printing medication reports from the HosXp system, allowing the small drug warehouse to withdraw drugs from the large one. Previously, balances were calculated on a weekly basis, followed by the issuance of a bill of lading to withdraw medicine from the large warehouse.
3. Adjust the product replenishment process using maximum and minimum values (max–min), instead of the previous method, which did not specify replenishment quantities. The disbursement method now occurs every four weeks, requiring the drug warehouse to notify the remaining balance rather than the amount needed to be disbursed.
4. Designate the large drug warehouse as the operator responsible for product replenishment at service points or drug depots. This way, the main medicine warehouse knows the balance from the small medicine warehouse, allowing the large pharmaceutical warehouse to replenish the agreed quantity.
5. Use the Visual Sign Control technique to mark the drug warehouse's shelves with maximum and minimum stock levels. This helps officials accurately assess stock levels and make correct purchasing decisions. Previously, shelves lacked labels, and officials relied on the Stock Card to gauge the balance, which sometimes led to discrepancies due to recording errors.

D.1.3 *Operation results*

1. Decreased the number of medicines kept at service and distribution points to minimize the issue of expired medicines and reduce medication withdrawals outside scheduled times.
2. To meet demand, maintain a sufficient reserve of drugs at service points and dispensing points.
3. Facilitate the withdrawal of medicine from a large medicine warehouse and support more frequent drug withdrawal cycles.
4. Minimize the use of product picking slips.
5. Conserve resources, personnel, time, and transportation at the service point, leading to higher officer satisfaction.
6. Procure the correct amount of medicine with increased accuracy.
7. Decrease risks associated with staff errors.

D.2 *Project: Develop and improve the hospital linen management system*

D.2.1 *Basic information and problem conditions (Figure 7.3)*

1. The workflow is redundant, as there are many steps involved in the fabric counting process.
2. The procedure for counting used contaminated cloth does not adhere to disease control principles. This includes a lack of data recording or the presence of incorrect records. This issue hinders effective data analysis.
3. Cloth resource allocation is based on experience and predictions, which sometimes results in more fabric than necessary. This leads to product hoarding. Conversely, there are instances of fabric shortages, indicating an imbalance between demand and the amount of fabric in reserve.

D.2.2 *Improvement strategies*

1. Determine the fabric quantity level using maximum and minimum values (max–min) for effective control of use and withdrawal.

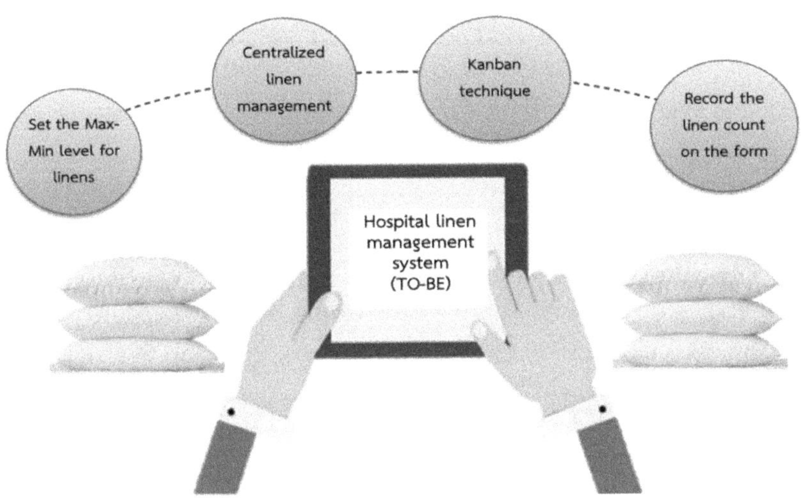

Figure 7.3. Improvement strategies for the hospital linen management system.

2. Implement centralized fabric management (Centralization).
3. Improve fabric management using the Kanban technique.
4. Establish a method to monitor the quantity of fabric associated with the patient and the amount of fabric that is damaged. Record data about fabric attached to the patient in a specified form, and set a framework for counting fabric, with a requirement for monthly counts. This will allow us to verify the quantity of fabric, type, and usage conditions.

D.2.3 *Operational results*

1. Minimizes risks associated with inadequate laundry supply at service points.
2. Encourages resource-sharing between agencies.
3. Enhances cloth management efficiency by providing clarity on the amount used in the hospital. This information can be utilized for further analysis.
4. Improves counting efficiency, reduces the time from three hours to just one hour, and ensures safety in the infection control laundry unit.
5. Enables root-cause analysis through data recording, allowing for immediate problem-solving and reducing complaints about torn or insufficient cloth.

D.3 *Project: Reduce the number of re-sterilizations of sterile medical supplies*

D.3.1 *Basic information and problem conditions*

1. Some service units store more sterile medical supplies than necessary, while others have shortages.
2. Sterile medical supplies are kept in several locations. Consequently, staff in each service unit are tasked with counting products and checking for expired items.
3. Under the current management system, it is currently impossible to utilize equipment on a first-in, first-out (FIFO) basis.

D.3.2 *Improvement strategies*

1. The quantity of sterile medical supplies is determined using the maximum and minimum values (max–min) of each type of equipment, and labels are created for communication among relevant officials.

2. Centralized equipment management allows sharing between service units. Equipment for sterilization is organized by type rather than by service unit.
3. Equipment must be returned three days before its expiration date so that it can be used by other units.
4. Equipment with low usage rates, but still necessary, should be packed in an additional plastic envelope to extend its lifespan from two weeks to six months.
5. Technology, such as LINE groups, should be used to facilitate communication between related personnel. Officials can send images and messages to inform relevant units about equipment nearing expiration, enabling immediate recycling and usage where needed.

D.3.3 *Operation results*

1. The risk of insufficient sterile medical supplies to meet demand is reduced.
2. The quantity of sterile medical supplies is appropriately matched to the amount used.
3. Redundant work steps are reduced, and the number of expired sterile medical supplies decreases by 86% within six months.
4. Storage space is reduced.
5. Resource sharing between units reduces various workloads.

E. Hospital E (Hospital size: 121 beds)

This is a sizable general hospital, boasting 201 beds, located in the eastern part of Bangkok. Recognized as a leading private international hospital, it offers general medical examination services. As of 2017, the hospital employs 574 staff members, comprising 177 doctors, 140 professional nurses, and 14 pharmacists, among others.

E.1 ***Project: Reduce re-sterilization and develop the central sterile services department (CSSD) system based on logistics principles***

E.1.1 *Basic information and problem conditions*

1. The reservation and distribution of medical equipment are managed manually without a computer system.
2. The rate at which medical materials are returned for re-sterilization is high.

3. The value of medical material reserves in the CSSD warehouse is uncertain and difficult to verify.
4. An effective system for inspecting and tracking the flow of medical equipment is lacking.
5. A single item of medical equipment has multiple names in the database system, making it impossible to know the actual quantity of medical equipment.

E.1.2 *Improvement strategies*

1. Create a database system to categorize all available medical equipment in the department. Assign one name to each item and define the product structure. Formulate sets of medical equipment with many items for a detailed breakdown.
2. The system should accurately record the quantity of all medical equipment in the central distribution department.
3. Set a selling price for each piece of medical equipment in the department, to enable cost calculation for the various parts involved.

E.1.3 *Operation results*

1. In the central distribution department, the value of medical equipment reserves has decreased.
2. The central disbursement department operates such as a warehouse, with the ability to check the quantity and items of inventory value through a computer system.
3. The cost of re-sterilizing tools on a daily basis has decreased.
4. Payment and equipment usage per patient can be accurately tracked.
5. The central distribution department can use the daily sales data to evaluate the adequacy of each tool's reserve and maintain the right amount.

F. Hospital F (850 beds)

Hospital F is located in the Mueang District, Chonburi Province, and is a government-run tertiary hospital with 850 beds. It provides services to a total population of 53,115 people, offering medical treatment across all fields of medicine and public health at tertiary, secondary, and primary medical care levels. It caters to outpatients, inpatients, and the general public. The hospital network includes 17 district health promotion hospitals and 1 branch hospital. Currently, the hospital employs 2,675 staff, which includes 220 doctors, 20 dentists, 696 professional nurses, 50 pharmacists, and other staff members (as of 2016).

F.1 *Project: Improving the efficiency of parcel management for medical materials*

F.1.1 *Basic information and problem conditions*

1. The procurement process involves extensive documentation and numerous approval steps, resulting in a lengthy ordering process that is sometimes delayed, leading to potential supply shortages. The lack of inventory level information across various units makes forecasting and purchase planning challenging, sometimes resulting in overstocking or shortages.
2. The warehouse storage space is inadequate for the quantity of products, leading to improper storage that does not meet standards.
3. Some types of parcels experience little to no movement, resulting in dead stock. When stored, the lack of clear signage indicating their location makes searching or verification time-consuming.
4. Warehouse management has been found to include duplicate information in the product list card (stock card), the Electronic Government Procurement (EGP) warehouse system, and the EPhis system, resulting in reduced efficiency.
5. The two information systems, the EPhis system and the EGP warehouse system, have been found to lack data connectivity. Various picking units record parcel pick-up requests through the EPhis system and send this information online to the warehouse. The warehouse then debits the required amount from the system, which must be paid for within the EGP warehouse system. As a result, the warehouse is unable to see the quantity of products available in subwarehouses or at the picking units, making it impossible to know the total amount of materials in the system. Furthermore, the information is not linked to which agency has withdrawn it, where it has been used, or for which patients. This lack of precision affects the data analysis.

6. Various hospital requisition units request supplies based on their needs and experience without clear guidelines, resulting in either a shortage or a surplus of supplies.
7. The absence of a clear timeframe for package pickup, along with a large number of withdrawal units (141 in total), can lead to work errors due to the rush to process simultaneous pickups.
8. Different picking units come to collect the parcel themselves, resulting in a loss of time and manpower.

F.1.2 *Improvement strategies*

1. Choose the types of medical materials and pilot units. The details of this step are as follows:
   - Use the ABC Analysis, discussed in Chapter 2 technique to select Type A medical materials, which are high-value groups, for the pilot project (as shown in Table 7.2).
   - Select pilot units. These are the wards that use the largest number of medical supplies. The goal is to reduce the amount of inventory in that unit, and then extend the results to all other wards.
2. Set the amount of product storage to match the actual usage rate. This involves letting the agency determine the minimum stock (3 days) and maximum stock (7–10 days), which were previously unspecified. The agencies can then withdraw materials as needed.
3. Develop the material delivery system as follows:
   - For external agencies and the warehouse: Use drop-shipping methods (e.g., Lab solutions, patient drinking water, garbage bags) to reduce warehouse space and costs.
   - For the supplies warehouse and various agencies: Change from the agencies picking up materials from the warehouse to the

Table 7.2. Classification of medical materials using the ABC analysis technique.

Medical Materials	Value (baht)	Quantity (items)
Type A	50,179,557	79
Type B	9,538,449	74
Type C	3,157,851	154

warehouse delivering materials using the VMI (Vendor Managed Inventory) system. This entails the warehouse controlling and replenishing materials when stocks drop to an agreed-upon level, as well as using the Milk Run transportation method for distribution.

4. Enhance and improve the parcel management information system. This involves updating the warehouse management program to link data on the quantity of goods picked and disbursed so that various disbursement units can record transactions and warehouse staff can view these transactions and see the balance and movement of medical supplies each day.
5. Design a new process for disbursing medical supplies. In the past, various agencies withdrew materials according to their needs without any control over the amount. The parcel officer deducted the payment from the number of items required by the agency and printed disbursement reports from the program. They then organized all of the materials according to the bill and notified various agencies to pick them up at the warehouse. The new process begins with checking the system's balances in various departments. The system records the withdrawal of medical supplies from the department when the remaining supplies reach the predetermined minimum level. Payments are withdrawn from the system based on the amount disbursed. Medical supplies are then arranged according to the requested list and delivered to the agency.

F.1.3 *Operation results*

1. Procurement officers can use the system to check the quantities of materials across various departments. They can identify when the remaining quantity has reached the set minimum level and prepare to replenish materials according to the set maximum level.
2. The cost of holding medical supplies across all wards has been reduced. Initially, in fiscal year 2016, the hospital had an average monthly material disbursement value of 3,348,360 baht. Following the project implementation, this value decreased to an average of 2,854,155 baht per month, a reduction of 14.85%, as shown in Table 7.3.
3. The project also resulted in a reduction in travel time and costs. Initially, in fiscal year 2016, each ward would collect parcels from the depot, taking an average of 30 minutes each time. This

Table 7.3. Average material withdrawal value before and after project implementation.

Evaluate of the Decrease in the Value of Medical Materials Due to System Adjustments Across All Wards			
	Fiscal Year 2016	October 2016	Percentage of Reduced Value (%)
Average monthly material withdrawal value	3,348,360	2,854,155	14.85

Table 7.4. Comparison of transportation time and costs before and after project implementation.

	September 2016	October 2016	Percentage of Time Reduced (%)
Average transit time per month	9,450 minutes	2,880 minutes	69.52
Average monthly transportation costs (*)	22,491 baht	9,450 baht	69.52

Note: Staff wages are calculated at 20,000 baht per month and work for 7 hours with a 1-hour break; Working hours are from 8:30 a.m.–4:30 p.m., Monday to Saturday.

amounted to 9,450 minutes per month, or a cost of 22,491 baht. However, with the warehouse project implementation and the use of the Milk Run transportation system, this time was reduced to 2,880 minutes per month. The cost also decreased to 9,450 baht, a reduction of 69.52%, as shown in Table 7.4.

G. Hospital G (community hospital with 38 beds)

Hospital G is a community hospital with 30 beds, providing health services to people in the Sri Narong District of Surin Province and nearby districts. It also supports the service network of six subdistrict health promotion hospitals. Initially, the hospital served only outpatients and emergency accident patients within business hours. However, in January 2014, it expanded its services to include disease-specific clinics that operate every day, including public holidays, twenty-four hours a day. The hospital has a staffing capacity of

100 people, including 4 doctors, 2 dentists, 3 pharmacists, 23 registered nurses, and others. It serves a population of 4,203 people (information from 2018).

G.1 *Project: Master's Program in logistics, pharmaceutical inventory management, and medical material warehouse management*

G.1.1 *Basic information and problem conditions*

Currently, the hospital faces issues with expired medicines, dead stock medicines, and an oversupply of medical materials/saline due to unrealistic withdrawals. The hospital relies on experience and familiarity to deduct inventory in real time, using Excel for monthly inventory counts. There is a lack of stock control between the sub-drug warehouse and the drug room, leading to occasional medicine shortages before the withdrawal period.

G.1.2 *Improvement strategies*

1. The hospital addresses issues by analyzing work processes.
2. Data is collected by classifying drug groups using the ABC-VEN analysis technique.
3. Information systems are applied, starting with free platforms such as Google Sheets. This allows the ward staff to enter and update information, enabling the warehouse to access real-time data.

G.1.3 *Operation results*

1. Improved warehouse space management due to increased product turnover.
2. Reduced working hours (man-hours) in counting stock, leading to a more accurate drug value. This is because the drug inventory's value now aligns with the actual disbursement amount.

H. Hospital H (700 beds)

This hospital, located in Saraburi Province, offers high-quality, general public health services. It covers health promotion, disease prevention and control, medical treatment, and rehabilitation. The hospital is a high-level tertiary care center in five areas: cancer, accidents, cardiovascular disease, newborn care, and organ transplants. It supports a network of 27 subdistrict health promotion hospitals, two urban community public health centers, and four additional Saraburi hospitals under the Provincial Health Service Area Office. The hospital staff consists of 2,127 people, including 115 full-time doctors, 38 doctors in training (1st- and 3rd-year), 15 dentists, 40 pharmacists, and 564 professional nurses (data from 2018).

H.1 *Project: Development of internal VMI saline in hospitals*

H.1.1 *Basic information and problem conditions (Figure 7.4)*

1. The hospital identified a problem with the saline disbursement process. The current process is difficult and complicated, leading to waste, especially during the bill of lading, printing, and transport processes. As a result, employees make several trips, increasing operating costs.

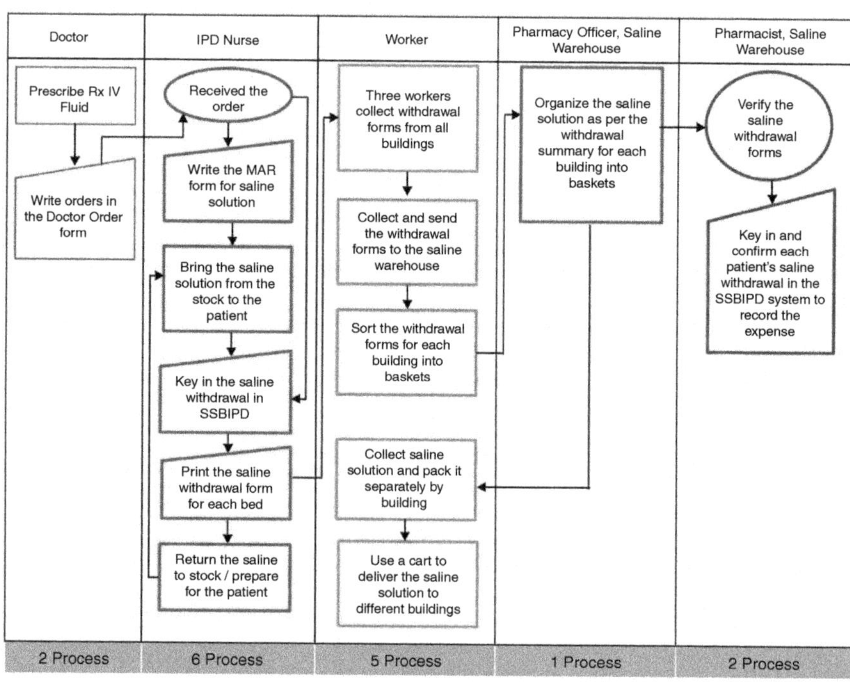

Figure 7.4. The saline disbursement process in hospital (AS-IS).

H.1.2 *Improvement strategies (Figure 7.5)*

1. Conduct a Business Process Analysis from the point of a doctor's order to the warehouse preparing products for delivery. The analysis identified several wasteful processes, which were then adjusted or eliminated, including

   - printing saline requisitions for each bed,
   - collecting requisitions from every building to deliver to the warehouse using three workers, and
   - confirming a saline requisition per person by logging into the SSB-IIPD system to calculate expenses.

2. Create a program that summarizes the saline withdrawal list by unit and modifies the saline confirmation system based on the data sent to the saline warehouse.

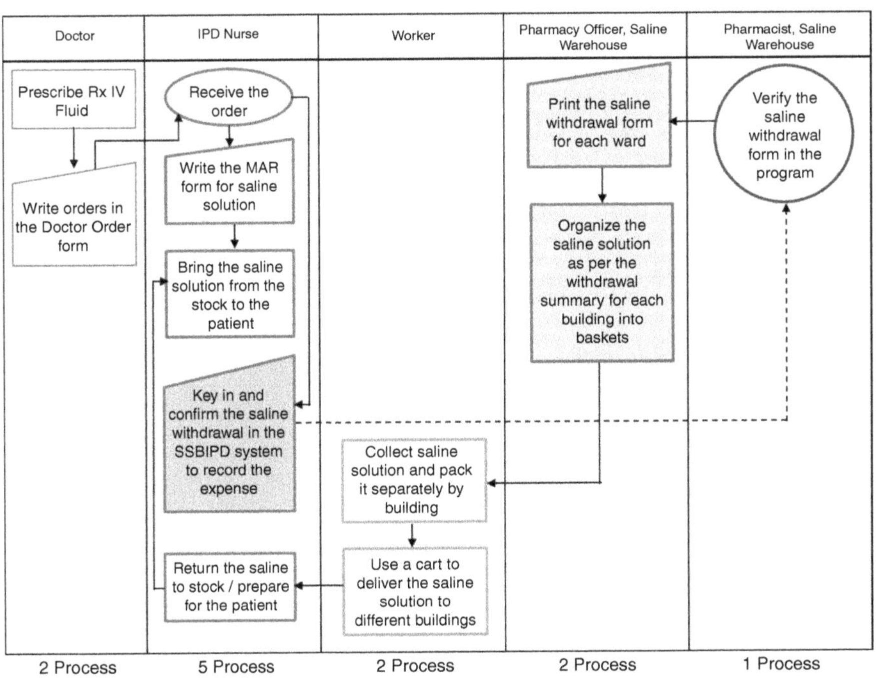

Figure 7.5. The saline disbursement process in hospital proposed.

3. Improve transportation by dividing the receiving-sending line by the amount of demand that occurs, divided into two periods: 8:30 a.m.–3:00 p.m. (split into three lines) and 3:00 p.m.–5:00 p.m. (one line).

H.1.3 *Operation results*

1. Reduced paper usage costs.
2. Reduced physical movement to pick up the bill of lading (only 56 meters per day).
3. Provided an overview of disbursements per ward, on one sheet.

H.2 *Project: Develop a drug inventory management system*

H.2.1 *Basic information and problem conditions*

1. At the end of the month, products from different companies are often sent together. This is because the hospital organizes ordering times so that they coincide. This causes congestion when waiting to receive products from companies that arrive at the same time, resulting in insufficient storage space.
2. Goods stored in the warehouse are unsorted, making it time-consuming to pick up or locate products.
3. When picking up products to prepare for payment, the picking unit does not follow the FIFO or First Expired, First Out (FEFO) order.
4. Sometimes, drugs are delivered to the wrong unit during transportation to the disbursement unit, and they are not always delivered on time.

H.2.2 *Improvement strategies*

1. Collect information about the types of medical supplies in each storage room.
2. Gather data on the number of medical supplies received and disbursed for each item.
3. To determine layout planning, study and collect information on the size of storage space, including images of the actual space.
4. Change the method of ordering products from once a month to distributing product orders daily. Consider the size and weight of the products and organize a system to determine the time period for

receiving medical supplies from the transport company to reduce congestion in transport vehicles.
5. Arrange the time for elevators used to transport medical supplies to and from warehouses.
6. Design a system for organizing bin locations by creating house numbers for products in the warehouse, making it convenient and easy to prepare products.
7. Adjust the process by having products arranged and checked to match the bill of lading before payment, to prevent mistakes in sending to the wrong agency, and to ensure the number is complete.

H.2.3 *Operation results*

1. This can reduce congestion in the warehouse area.
2. It makes product preparation more convenient and accurate.

I. Hospital I (community hospital with 60 beds)

This is a community hospital, Level F 2, with 60 beds. It provides health services to people in Chiang Saen, Chiang Rai Province, and nearby provinces, including public health services along the Lao Myanmar border. For outpatient services, the hospital serves an average of 12,060 people per month, while for inpatient services, it serves an average of 244 people per month. It also functions as a host hospital, supporting a service network of 13 subdistrict health promotion hospitals. Currently, the hospital has a total staff capacity of 236 people, including 7 doctors, 5 dentists, 6 pharmacists, 54 professional nurses, and others (data from 2018).

I.1 *Project: Supply chain management and pharmaceutical logistics for medical supplies (non-drugs) and general materials in hospitals and health service networks*

I.1.1 *Basic information and problem conditions*

The product disbursement system for hospitals and subdistrict health promotion hospitals in the areas for which the hospitals are responsible is not as efficient as it should be due to the following reasons:

1. There are more steps than necessary, leading to wasted time and waiting.

2. The programs used are diverse.
3. Database systems are different, making it impossible to link databases for joint systematic development.
4. Personnel must perform redundant tasks, increasing the workload.
5. The chance of errors is increased, leading to higher costs and not delivering as much value as it should deliver.

I.1.2 *Improvement strategies*

1. Modify the inventory management system to create a linkage of information between the warehouse and the point of use. The details of the adjustment are as follows:
   - Medicine warehouse: old system DRUG -> new system MMIS.
   - Central warehouse: old system, Napalai and Neo -> new system MMIS.
   - Cloth warehouse and drug distribution system DM/HT: old system Manual -> new system Electronic—QR Code.
2. Adjust logistics systems and warehouse supply chains: Adjust methods for sending bills of lading. By increasing the frequency of withdrawals and adjusting the process to reduce the waiting period after submitting the bill of lading.
3. Adjust methods, formats, and routes for transporting goods.
4. At the picking unit, reduce the product reserve rate.
5. Design additional programs to connect and send data from product ordering programs JHCIS (healthcare hospital) and PEED (financial, supplies, and plans).
6. Use ABC/VEN, Minimum Requirement, Just-in-Time, KANBAN, VMI systems.
7. Establish a central transportation system.
8. Adjust the document flow system, information, and parcel inspection.

I.1.3 *Operation results*

1. Enhance the value stream.
2. Minimize and reduce waste.
3. Decrease the value of inventory at the picking unit.
4. Lower transportation expenses in the product disbursement system.
5. Boost the satisfaction of service recipients.

J. Hospital J (924 beds)

This is a provincial hospital with a capacity of 1,022 beds, providing health services to people in Udon Thani Province and nearby provinces. The total population in the area of responsibility is approximately 5,545,010 people. The hospital's services are divided into outpatient services, which average 77,199 people per month, and inpatient services, which average 30,930 people per month. It is a host hospital for transferring high-level secondary and tertiary care in five areas: cardiology, cancer, newborn, trauma, and transplant. The hospital supports a service network of 32 subdistrict health promotion hospitals. Currently, the hospital has a total staffing capacity of 3,062 people, including 206 doctors, 18 dentists, 68 pharmacists, 1,081 professional nurses, and others (information from 2018).

J.1 *Project: Reduce congestion in waiting to receive medicine among outpatients*

J.1.1 *Basic information and problem conditions*

- The hospital faced issues with patient waiting times for medication, particularly for those with chronic diseases. This group significantly impacted the waiting times. It was observed that on Mondays, when only the clinic for patients with chronic diseases was operational, the average wait time for medication was two hours and five minutes. However, on Tuesdays, when an additional neurosurgery clinic was open, the wait time for medication increased during the same data collection period. The data indicated that on Tuesday, the waiting time was 1 hour and 52 minutes. However, if all patients were accounted for, it was found that the waiting time for medication extended until 8:00 p.m.–9:00 p.m., unlike Monday, which ended at 4:00 p.m. During the peak hours of 10:00 a.m.–1:00 p.m., the waiting time for medication remained the same. This may be because pharmacists and officials, aware of the increased patient load on Tuesdays, expedited medication dispensation more than usual.

J.1.2 *Improvement strategies*

1. Develop and improve the drug dispensing process by conducting business process analysis and using lean concepts to enhance the following:

- Eliminating unnecessary work (elimination) to increase speed and serve patients faster.
- Making work easier (simplification) to create a continuous flow for dispensing medicine, reducing wait time from 5 to 10 minutes to dispensing 3–5 queues at a time by adding drug dispensing channels from 2 to 3 (rotate manpower on Monday, Tuesday, and Wednesday).
- If there is a large number of patients using the service in the morning and the available resources are insufficient, adjustments will be made by increasing the auxiliary workforce in the afternoon.

2. Develop a joint drug dispensing unit with private pharmacies and other government dispensing units. Design a drug dispensing system using a drug program to connect data and provide co-dispensing units for drug stores in Udon Municipality.

J.1.3 *Operation results*

Prescribing medicine for patients with chronic diseases such as diabetes, high blood pressure, and heart disease reduced the waiting time for medicine by approximately 50–60%.

K. Hospital K (600 beds)

Hospital K is a provincial hospital with a capacity of 600 beds, serving the Mueang Samut Prakan District and managing referrals from all hospital networks. Each day, we see a growing number of patients, with an average of 2,405 individuals seeking outpatient services. Its bed occupancy rate often exceeds capacity, reaching 124%. The hospital employs a dedicated team of 1,441 staff members.

K.1 *Project: Streamline operations, centralize transport, transition to digital patient records*

K.1.1 *Basic information and problem conditions*

The hospital deploys logistics expertise to address five issues.

1. The transportation of prescriptions, medicines, and specimens remains inefficient.
2. The retrieval of patient histories is time-consuming due to a lack of control systems in the data collection process. The average time

for this process is 60 per list, often because patient names cannot be located.
3. Personnel exhibit gaps in knowledge regarding material system management, leading to errors such as incorrect product or quantity selection.
4. The excessive paperwork involved is evidence of overproduction.
5. Overstocking is a concern with material storage exceeding necessary quantities.

K.1.2 *Improvement strategies*

1. The hospital has formed a central logistics team for the efficient collection and delivery of prescriptions, medicines, and specimens. This aligns with the concept of centralization and the pull resource principle, with a pick-up and drop-off scheduled every half hour to prevent backlog.
2. The hospital has embraced lean process improvements, leveraging information technology systems for efficiency, thereby reducing paper use.
3. The use of E-Kanban minimizes the need for sending bills of lading, helps adjust the withdrawal cycle, creates visual control with Kanban, improves workflow per the 5S principle, and optimizes space usage by reducing or eliminating non-beneficial steps.
4. Work standards have been established, and training is provided to relevant personnel.

K.1.3 *Operation results*

1. Hospitals can reduce trips for walking and transporting drugs and specimens and increase the satisfaction of staff in each unit, ward staff, and pharmacy staff.
2. Hospitals can reduce the time to access patient history and reduce patient waiting time.
3. The value of material inventories decreased by 66%.
4. There are no instances where materials will expire in the warehouse.
5. The hospital is able to reduce the entire process time by 72.84% (from the original 13 steps to only 7 steps).

L. Hospital L (80 beds)

This community hospital, located in Buriram Province, has 90 beds and provides health services to the public in Khu Mueang District and adjacent districts. On average, the hospital provides 10,484 outpatient and 417 inpatient services per month. It also functions as a quality host hospital, supporting a network of 10 subdistrict health promotion hospitals. The hospital currently has a staff capacity of 227 staff numbers, including 8 doctors, 5 dentists, 9 pharmacists, and 57 professional nurses, among others (data as of 2018).

L.1 *Project: Logistics with inventory/warehouse management and transportation of essential medicine to Subdistrict Health Promoting Hospitals*

L.1.1 *Basic information and problem conditions*

1. Warehouse management of medical materials/non-drug supplies is currently inefficient due to overstocking. This is because officials do not know the exact usage amount, and there is no precise forecast. Orders are placed based on previous experience.
2. The transportation of essential medicine to the 10 subdistrict health promotion hospitals in the network is costly. Each hospital must travel every two months to submit a requisition and then travel again 10 days later to receive the medicine. Additionally, subdistrict health promotion hospitals also face issues with expired medicines and off-cycle withdrawals.

L.1.2 *Improvement strategies*

1. The hospital has revamped its product management program by separating groups of medical materials/non-drug supplies based on value according to ABC principles.
2. Kanban is introduced to assist with product counting in both warehouses and wards and to adjust withdrawal amounts according to actual usage as indicated on the Kanban sheet. The method of replenishing items has also been adjusted from ward-responsible withdrawals to warehouse-managed replenishments.
3. The principles of the Traveling Salesman Problem are applied to arrange routes for medicine transportation to subdistrict health promotion hospitals. Delivery is divided into two zones: northern and southern. The hospital alternates delivery between these zones and adds an online communication channel to notify of disbursement rounds at the end of every month.

L.1.3 *Operation results*

1. Hospitals can reduce inventory costs and free up more space in warehouses.
2. We can increase the level of satisfaction and improve the efficiency in allocating drugs to subdistrict health promotion hospitals. This means that Subdistrict Health Promotion Hospitals receive medicines on the specified date, off-cycle drug withdrawals are reduced, and the time and cost of transporting medicines are decreased (reducing gas costs by 36%). There will be no overdue or incorrect medication payments, and time loss for personnel arriving to receive medication will be reduced.

M. Hospital M (600 beds)

This is a provincial hospital with a capacity of 520 beds, providing health services to people in Phrae Province and nearby provinces. The hospital serves an average of 1,934 outpatients and 3,113 inpatients per month. It also acts as a host hospital, supporting a service network of 29 subdistrict health promotion hospitals. Currently, the hospital has a total staffing capacity of 1,480 people, including 100 doctors, 504 dentists, 11 pharmacists, 40 professional nurses, and others (information as of 2018).

M.1 *Project: Management of warehouses, materials, medical supplies, drugs, and central transportation systems*

M.1.1 *Basic information and problem conditions*

1. Identified problems with inventory management of consumables, saline, medical materials, tools, and re-sterilized items, such as the issue of stocking more products than necessary. This leads to an overstock of products, causing them to deteriorate or expire prematurely. There is also a problem with not knowing the inventory status of the main warehouse and subwarehouse.

M.1.2 *Improvement strategies*

1. Conduct an assessment of the use of consumables and collect data every month. Once the data are analyzed, adjust the fixed stock amount for each department to be sufficient and appropriate.

2. To manage saline inventory, use the Kanban Card and barcode system. This is to determine the total inventory of saline within the hospital.
3. Use the inventory program to manage medical material inventory. This is to create a link between the front office and back-office systems (back office).
4. Establish a central transportation agency to make the central distribution unit's transportation system more efficient. Organize rounds and routes for transporting re-sterile tools to various departments in the hospital.

M.1.3 *Operation results*

1. Consumable products have sufficient and appropriate inventory. The inventory value decreased by 40%.
2. Saline products have sufficient and appropriate amounts. The amount of saline withdrawn from the system (patient expenses) equals the amount of saline withdrawn from the warehouse.
3. Medical material products have a sufficient and appropriate inventory. The inventory value decreased by 7%.
4. There has been a decrease in the quantity of re-sterile and sterile tool products in various departments, along with a reduction in the time and distance of transportation.

N. Hospital N (252 beds)

Hospital N is a general hospital with 252 beds, providing healthcare services to the population in Tha Maka District, Kanchanaburi Province, and nearby districts. On average, we provide outpatient services to 28,771 individuals and inpatient services to 1,318 individuals per month. We are also a referral hospital for secondary and tertiary care, supporting a network of 15 subdistrict health promotion hospitals. At present, our hospital team consists of 694 staff members, including 36 doctors, 11 dentists, 19 pharmacists, 245 professional nurses, and other professionals (as per 2018 data).

N.1 *Project: Development of central transport agency and material inventory management*

N.1.1 *Basic information and problem conditions*

1. An issue with inventory management has been identified, stemming from the process of withdrawing medical supplies based on

estimates rather than data analysis. This practice results in overstocking and, consequently, increased storage costs.

2. The hospital's internal goods transport system is inefficient. Each department's housekeeping staff independently retrieves products from various warehouses, leading to resource wastage in terms of manpower, time, and cost.

N.1.2 *Improvement strategies*

1. The ABC analysis technique should be used to determine the quantity of medical supply reserves. This approach involves grouping products according to their importance and adjusting the withdrawal cycle accordingly. Furthermore, techniques for determining the appropriate reorder point should be implemented.
2. A central transportation agency should be established, utilizing the Milk Run technique for the delivery of various goods—including cloth, medical supplies, CSSD, medicines, parcels, saline, and hemodialysis fluid—to different departments within the hospital.

N.1.3 *Operation results*

1. Adequate and sufficient supply of medical items, reducing the inventory value by 53%.
2. The establishment of a central transportation agency resulted in a 46% decrease in transportation time, a 35% decrease in transportation costs, a 91% decrease in transportation personnel, and a 47% decrease in transportation cycles.

O. Hospital O (601 beds)

This hospital is a high-level tertiary institution with the potential to provide comprehensive treatment in all fields. It serves as a transfer point for patients from other hospitals, offering a variety of services to outpatients, inpatients, and emergency patients across all specialties. It hosts various centers of excellence, such as the Heart Center, Stroke Center, Level-1 Trauma Center, Eye Disease Center, and Comprehensive Kidney Replacement Center. In addition to this, it serves as an institution for students from the Faculty of Medicine to teach, research, and practice. The hospital has a total staff capacity of 2,638, including 227 full-time doctors, 16 dentists, 39 pharmacists, 778 professional nurses, and others (2018 data).

O.1 *Project: Management of medical supply warehouses with a barcode system*

O.1.1 *Basic information and problem conditions*

1. The procedure for disbursing medical supplies involves many complicated steps, making it impossible for the agency to specify its use and analyze the data to find an appropriate reserve rate for the warehouse.
2. Counting the organization's balance is challenging.
3. An error occurred in the navigation process for medical supplies for patients, resulting in inadequate cost recovery.

O.1.2 *Improvement strategies*

1. The hospital has studied product group information and used ABC analysis principles for consideration. This is to classify product groups and select which ones are appropriate for barcode sticker installation. The result is a list of medical supplies priced at 100 baht and up.
2. Create an internal database to store master data for medical supplies that will be used in the barcode system.
3. Design and adjust new work processes. The printing and pasting of barcode stickers are the next step. This will be incorporated into the warehouse receipt process.
4. Other logistics concepts include adjusting ordering methods by taking lead time information into account and adjusting the product replenishment process each time by setting maximum and minimum values (max–min).

O.1.3 *Operation results*

1. The barcode system helps various departments work more conveniently. Errors in disbursement are reduced.
2. The value of withdrawing medical supplies has decreased.

O.2 *Project: Develop the central transportation agency*

O.2.1 *Basic information and problem conditions*

A hospital has a total of 115 departments inside the hospital and 3 departments outside the hospital. The transportation system is separate for pick-up and delivery by the ward or department, sending the housekeeper or clerk of each department to pick up various products. These include inventory, cloth, CSSD, medical materials, medicine, and medical supplies, which are located in different places according to each product type. Each time, the housekeeper or clerk must take time to walk, wait for the elevator, and wait to receive the goods. This takes about 30–40 minutes each time, resulting in wasted resources in terms of personnel, time, and costs.

O.2.2 *Improvement strategies (Figure 7.6)*

1. Establish a central transportation agency (pull resource). By centralizing agencies together with stretcher services in transportation and using the Milk Run transportation technique, the central transportation agency will be responsible for transporting various products, including cloth, medical supplies, parcels, and specialized medical supplies, to all departments within and outside the hospital.
2. Improve the information system to create links between purchasing work and various departments throughout the hospital.

O.2.3 *Operation results*

1. The time spent on receiving and sending tools, clothing, medical supplies, office supplies, and specialized medical supplies now takes 35% less time. Personnel have reduced the time spent on receiving and sending tools, cloth, medical supplies, office supplies, and specialized medical supplies (20%).
2. The unit received the products more completely and quickly. The unit's satisfaction level has increased.

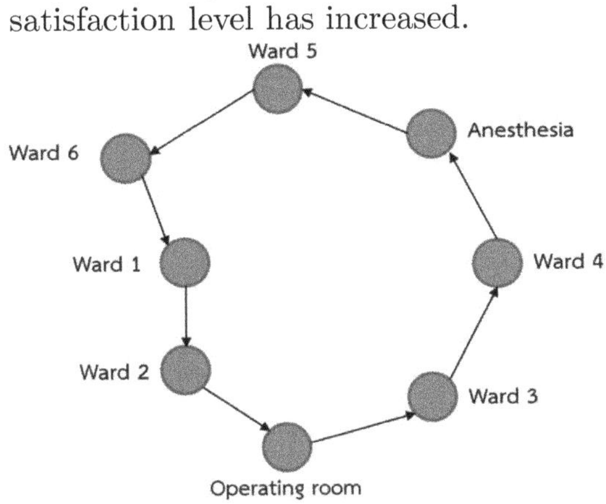

Figure 7.6. A central transportation agency utilizing the Milk Run transportation technique (pull resource).

P. Hospital P (875 beds)

The hospital is located in Bangkok and has a capacity of 1,000 beds. The hospital has a total staff of 1,967 members, including 304 full-time doctors, 15 dentists, 49 pharmacists, 1,019 professional nurses, and others (2018 data).

P.1 *Project: Improving the efficiency of drug distribution in the central receiving-delivery unit*

P.1.1 *Basic information and problem conditions*

— Before joining the project, the hospital had transported medicines via the central transportation agency. However, there were inefficiencies in the transportation system. For instance, it took a long time to transport medicine from the dispensary to the ward, and the medicine was often damaged during transportation. Late start times resulted in hasty work without proper checks. Additionally, shared resources (people and carts) were not considered, leading to wasted resources in terms of people, time, and costs.

P.1.2 *Improvement strategies*

1. Increase the work efficiency of staff by improving the work process for recording working time and adjust the working hours of staff to ensure they start work faster, including modifying the medicine dispensing unit to pack medication into bags in advance.
2. Increase transportation efficiency by changing transportation methods using the Milk Run technique and dividing transportation cycles into similar areas. This includes documenting the delivery time at each point to analyze the data and enhance efficiency.

P.1.3 *Operation results*

1. When comparing incident reports from three months before and after the change to pre-packing drugs in bags at the inpatient pharmacy, it was found that instances of broken drugs decreased from ten to two, and missing drugs decreased from two to one.
2. After collecting data from the time of dispensing drugs to evaluate the results of adjusting the method of packing drugs in bags, it was found that the waiting time to receive drugs from the central receiving unit was reduced from forty minutes per ward to no more than ten minutes.

3. Data collected from nursing staff's work time records revealed that nurses had more time to check drugs, and the number of drugs sent to the wrong wards was reduced.

7.2 Executive-Level Perspectives on the Importance of Logistics Systems in Hospitals

7.2.1 *University Hospital A*

The hospital has introduced the Lean concept to improve and develop the hospital's internal resources and processes. To solve the problem of congestion and service delays that cause bottleneck processes, another important issue is the problem of transportation within the hospital. At present, each unit has separate transportation; different people carry different things, resulting in a high workload at any one time, which causes delays. The hospital addresses this issue by establishing pick-up and drop-off points within the building, which subsequently collect and transport the items to various agencies. The hospital addresses this issue by establishing pick-up and drop-off points within the building, which subsequently collect and transport the items to various agencies.

Inventory issues arise from the problem of keeping more stock than necessary. This is because officials pick up products according to expectations, resulting in expired goods and storage costs. Currently, we are addressing this issue by implementing automatic machines, such as vending machines, to store products for use in the Emergency Department (ER). This allows for control over product replenishment when usage reaches a predetermined threshold.

And finally, the hospital has a plan to develop an automatic medication management system with a radio frequency identification (RFID) system to reduce human error. Being able to administer medication at the specified time helps reduce the workload of the operator and increases efficiency in providing patient services.

7.2.2 *University Hospital B*

The hospital has developed an information system to create a link between the main warehouse and various subwarehouses. This is accomplished by applying a barcode system to medical materials in each hospital unit. Bar code stickers are attached at the item level to track hospital medical supplies through the process of receiving them into the warehouse, disbursing them, and providing services to patients.

The factors that drive success in the project are as follows:

1. Senior executives must understand the importance of buy-in and take the initiative to support the project.
2. Stakeholder involvement and participation from relevant agencies need to be incorporated into the project from the beginning.
3. Committees and working groups should be set up.
4. Once trained, the quick win project should be implemented immediately and not be delayed.
5. Once the problem has been solved, it should be set as a standard, or Objectives and Key Results (OKR), for measurement and evaluation within the organization.

7.2.3 *University Hospital C*

The hospital can apply logistics principles to solve problems in three areas, as follows:

1. Drug warehouse management problems, which include issues with disbursement and control of drug use in the ward. The hospital has designed a drug unit conversion system to facilitate usage recording. This results in more accurate drug stocking, and improvements have been made in medication transportation. The design incorporates designated zones for transportation, thereby minimizing distance and time.
2. Management of medical material warehouses is a significant issue in hospitals. Many departments use medical materials, resulting in a large number of storage or backup nodes. Especially in the Operating Room (OR) department, the problem is that stock is stored in large quantities, and it is not possible to know the current quantity or usage amount. As a result, the problem was solved by dissolving unnecessary nodes and implementing a system for recording disbursements. This includes guidelines for solving future problems using barcode techniques.
3. Problems with the carpool system include delayed service due to walking around looking for a stretcher. The number of stretchers and staff is insufficient. The hospital has improved by adjusting the location of the new wheelchair equipment, adjusting staffing

levels accordingly (resource allocation), and having various agencies record requests for the use of stretchers. This data is used to analyze and prioritize work distribution. As a result of this project's implementation, the problem of timely service was greatly reduced.

7.3 Transfer the Lessons Learned to Factors of Success in the Project

After visiting the area and taking part in research studies, which included interviews with people involved at all levels, from the operational to the executive level, the project's success factors can be summed up in six points:

1. **Top Management Support:** Executives must have a clear vision for organizational development. This is an important first step that will lead to positive change. Furthermore, executives must be influential in stimulating personnel to see the importance of project creation.
2. **Strong Organizational Culture (Strong Culture):** Personnel understand the importance of quality development and actively cooperate.
3. **Communication and User Involvement:** There is communication within and between departments. Teamwork occurs in the organization, and work is done together to form a cross-functional team.
4. **Learn to Analyze Data (Fact Analysis):** Performance is measured and evaluated using OKR (Objective & Key Results) and KPI (Key Performance Indicators) techniques as a driving force for developing work to be more efficient.
5. **Using Information Technology as a Tool for Knowledge Management:** This includes having clear goals and operational plans.
6. **End-to-End Process Method to Solve Problems:** Problems are addressed by analyzing and improving the entire system or process. If only one process is modified, the problem is passed on to the next. Ultimately, the issue will persist, preventing any genuine improvement or development.

7.4 Conclusion

The final chapter synthesized lessons from previous sections to present best practices for hospital logistics. These include standardization of processes, integration of digital systems, and resilience planning to withstand disruptions. Case studies from Thailand demonstrated how pilot projects can be scaled up to improve service delivery across multiple hospitals. The emphasis throughout the chapter was that best practices are not static—they must be adapted to the size, resources, and needs of individual hospitals.

The lesson here is that patient safety and service quality remain the ultimate measures of logistics success. Logistics is not just about efficiency but also about creating systems that support high-quality care under all conditions. Hospitals that embrace continuous improvement and localized adaptation of best practices will not only optimize their logistics but also strengthen their role in delivering better healthcare outcomes for their communities and ultimately enhance overall health system performance.

Bibliography

Bowersox, D. J., Closs, D. J., & Cooper, M. B. (2012). *Supply Chain Logistics Management* (4th ed.). McGraw-Hill Education.

Chalermchon, W. (2010). The global GS1 traceability standard: Global standard for traceability systems [in Thai]. Department of Primary Industries and Mines. http://www.dpim.go.th/service/download?articleid=321&F=351.

Chanpuypetch, W. & Kritchanchai, D. (2015). An empirical-based construction of the multi-purpose process reference model for hospital supply chain. *Industrial Engineering, Management Science and Applications, 349*, 901–912.

Chanpuypetch, W. & Kritchanchai, D. (2017). A Design thinking framework and design patterns for hospital pharmacy management. *International Journal of Healthcare Management.* https://doi.org/10.1080/20479700.2017.1389479.

Chanpuypetch, W. & Kritchanchai, D. (2018). A process reference model for hospital supply chain of pharmaceutical products. *Industrial Engineering and Management System, 17*(1), 43–61. https://doi.org/10.7232/iems.2018.17.1.043.

Charupat, O. & Chaowalitwong, P. (2013). Heuristic for open vehicle routing to reduce transportation costs. *Engineering Journal, 4*(3), 45–55. https://www.ej.eng.chula.ac.th/.

Din, K., Kritchanchai, D., & Dokkulab, A. (2019). Time-driven activity-based costing in outpatient logistics. In *Proceedings of the International Conference on Industrial Engineering and Operations Management* (pp. 5–7). Bangkok, Thailand.

Engel Seth, P., White, B. E., Mundal Trude, I., Eines, F., & Kritchanchai D. (2020). Systems modelling to support the complex nature of healthcare services. *International Journal of Health and Technology*. https://doi.org/10.1007/s12553-020-00504-8.

GS1. (2013). *Global Traceability Standard for Healthcare (GTSH): Business Process and System Requirements for Supply Chain Traceability GS1 Standard*. http://www.gs.org/docs/gsmp/traceability/Global_Traceability_Standard_Healthcare.pdf.

Jiraporn, L., *et al.* (2011). *Development of a National Drug Database and an Internet-Based Search System for Effective Supply Chain Linkage and Improved Public Safety* [in Thai]. Thailand Research Fund, Thailand.

Jüttner, U., Christopher, M., & Godsell, J. (2010). A strategic framework for integrating marketing and supply chain strategies. *The International Journal of Logistics Management, 21*(1), 104–126. https://doi.org/10.1108/09574091011042213.

Kanjanapachara, T., Kaewman, T., Jongsomsuk, N., Kritchanchai, D., & Wasusri, T. (2024). Designing approaches to manage medicine and medical supply warehouses using a distribution center. In *The Conference of Industrial Engineering Network (IE NETWORK 2024) Proceedings* (pp. 1034–1036). Thai Industrial Engineering Association.

Kritchanchai, D. (2012). *Fact Sheet: National Drug Code and Database* [in Thai]. Mahidol University.

Kritchanchai, D., Doung, P., Khem, C., & Srisakunwan, S. Innovative practice and supply chain resilience during COVID-19 pandemic: A case study in Thailand. *The Impact of COVID-19 on Supply Chain Management*. https://doi.org/10.51432/978-1-8381524-2-0-5.

Kritchanchai, D., Engelseth, P., & Srisakunwan, S. (2018). Implementing and using new information technology in hospital logistics. In *2018 IEEE International Conference on Industrial Engineering and Engineering Management (IEEM)* (pp. 1186–1190). IEEE. https://doi.org/10.1109/IEEM.2018.8607865.

Kritchanchai, D., *et al.* (2011). *Application and Development of Hospital Logistics and Supply Chain Management: Case Study* [in Thai]. Mahidol University, Thailand.

Kritchanchai, D., *et al.* (2013). *Development of Electronic Data Exchange Systems in Healthcare Supply Chains* [in Thai]. Mahidol University, Thailand.

Kritchanchai, D., *et al.* (2015). *Research for the Development of Community Hospital Logistics Systems* [in Thai]. Thailand Research Fund, Thailand.

Kritchanchai, D., *et al.* (2016). *Research for Designing and Developing Infrastructure Logistics Systems, Information Integration, and Big*

Data Initiatives for Public Health in Thailand's Digital Economy [in Thai]. Thailand Research Fund, Thailand.

Kritchanchai, D. & Hoeur, S. (2017). Simulation modelling for facility allocation of outpatient department. *International Journal of Healthcare Management, 2017*. https://doi.org/10.1080/20479700.2017.1359920.

Kritchanchai, D., Hoeur, S., & Engelseth, P. (2018). Develop a strategy for improving healthcare logistics performance. *Supply Chain Forum: An International Journal, 19*(1), 2018. https://doi.org/10.1080/16258312.2017.1416876.

Kritchanchai, D. & Kritchanchai, S. (2016). Developing inventory management policy for drugs with medium and low consumption value in hospital. *Thai Pharmaceutical and Health Science Journal, 11*(4), 153–160.

Kritchanchai, D., Kritchanchai, S., Hoeur, S., & Tan, A. (2019). Healthcare supply chain management: Macro and micro perspectives. *Scientific Journal of Logistics LogForum, 15*(4), 531–544. https://doi.org/10.17270/J.LOG.2019.371.

Kritchanchai, D. & Meesamut, W. (2015). Developing inventory management in hospital. *International Journal of Supply Chain Management, 4*(2), 9–19.

Kritchanchai, D. & Muangchoo, S. (2013). *Healthcare Logistics and Supply Chain Management*. Mahidol University, Thailand.

Kritchanchai, D., Muangchoo, S., & Tan, A. (2019). Improving the efficiency of healthcare supply chain in Thailand. *International Journal of Electronic Healthcare, 4*, 313–329.

Kritchanchai, D., Senarak, D., Supeekit, T., & Chanpuypetch, W. (2024). Evaluating supply chain network models for third party logistics operated supply-processing distribution in Thai hospitals: An AHP-Fuzzy TOPSIS approach. *Logistics, 8*, 116. https://doi.org/10.3390/logistics8040116.

Kritchanchai, D., Somboonwiwat, T., & Chanpuypetch, W. (2015). Supply chain of Thailand product champion: A case study of the passenger car tire industry. *International Journal of Logistics Systems and Management, 20*, 83–102.

Kritchanchai, D., Srinon, R., Kietdumrongwong, P., Jansuwan, J., Phanuphak, N., & Chanpuypetch, W. (2024). Enhancing home delivery of emergency medicine and medical supplies through clustering and simulation techniques: A case study of COVID-19 home isolation in Bangkok. *Heliyon, 10*, e33177. https://doi.org/10.1016/j.heliyon.2024.e33177.

Kritchanchai, D. & Srisakunwan, S. (2023a). *Hospital Logistics Management*. LogHealth, Faculty of Engineering, Mahidol University, Thailand. (Adapted and expanded from the original work published in Thai as **การจัดการโลจิสติก ส์ในโรงพยาบาล**).

Kritchanchai, D., & Srisakunwan, S. (2023b). *Logistics and Supply Chain for Healthcare Operations Management.*

Kritchanchai, D., Thanakanjanaroj, M., Phanwongsal, S., Iamwattanasin, P., & Srisakunwan, S. (2021). Key success factor for manufacturer joint delivery system in modern trade. *SWU Engineering Journal, 16*(2), 16–27.

Kritchanchai, D., Wahab, S. N., Tan, A., & Mak, T., (2022). An analytical hierarchy process-based decision making for sustainable medical devices development. *LogForum 18*(4), 481–493. https://doi.org/10.17270/J.LOG.2022.768.

McKinsey & Company. (2012). *Strength in Unity: The Promise of Global Standards in Healthcare.*

Muangchoo, S. & Kritchanchai, D. (2015). National drug information sharing in the Thailand health care supply chain. *Therapeutic Innovation & Regulatory Science, 49*, 920–928.

Muangchoo, S., *et al.* (2013). *The Project for Traceability in Logistics and Supply Chain Management of Medicines.* National Research Council of Thailand and Thailand Research Fund, Thailand.

National Patient Safety Agency. (2007). *Safety in Doses: Medication Safety Incidents in the NHS.*

Niemsakul, J., Sardar, M., Islam, N., Singkarin, D., & Somboonwiwat, T. (2018). Cost-benefit sharing in healthcare supply chain collaboration. *International Journal of Logistics System and Management.* https://doi.org/10.1504/IJLSM.2018.10009326.

Piyawan, L. (2014). Patient safety and quality: Patient safety [in Thai]. The Healthcare Accreditation Institute. http://web.bcnpy.ac.th/bcnfile/index.php/bcnpy-risk?download=21:qa-to-quality-of-life.

Pujawan, N., Arief, M. M., Tjahjono, B., & Kritchanchai, D. (2015). An integrated shipment planning and storage capacity decision under uncertainty: A simulation study. *International Journal of Physical Distribution & Logistics Management, 45*, 913–937.

Ransikarbum, K., Kritchanchai, D., Chanpuypetch, W., & Niemsakul, J. (2024). Central hospital location and distribution planning using integrated K-Means and vehicle routing algorithm in the healthcare chain. *Operations and Supply Chain Management, 17*(2), 299–315.

Siriraj Foundation. (2021). *AI for Hospital's Demand Forecasting and Inventory Management: Medical and Non-Medical Products by Using 5G Networks* (Adapted). Bangkok, Thailand.

Sivaporn, S. & Tarinee, M. (2019). Reducing transportation costs by applying vehicle routing problem: A case study of an automotive parts distributor [in Thai]. *Kasem Bundit Engineering Journal, 9*(1), 1–10.

Srinon, R., Kritchanchai, D., Srisakunwan, S., & Kietdumrongwong, P. (2022). Policy brief-logistics and supply chain management strategy to support patient home isolation during the COVID-19 pandemic in Thailand. *Journal of the Medical Association of Thailand, 105*(11), 1160–1170.

Srinon, R., Kritchanchai, D., & Wasusri, T., International transport and Logistics of Vaccines Across Borders: The case of the Asia-Pacific Region, ARTNeT Working Paper Series No. 220 November 2022, Bangkok, ESCAP, http://hdl.handle.net/10419/266157.

Srisakunwan, S. & Petison, P. (2017). *A Study of the Pre-implementation Management Process for RFID Technology in Hospital Healthcare a Conceptual Paper*, London, UK, ICSSH, The 23rd ICSSH Conference.

Stock, J. R. & Lambert, D. M. (2001). *Strategic Logistics Management* (4th ed.). McGraw-Hill Irwin.

Supeekit, T., Somboonwiwat, T., & Kritchanchai, D. (2015). Linking hospital supply chain processes and performance to identify key performance indicator. *Industrial Engineering, Management Science and Applications, 349*, 927–938.

Walton, M., Woodward, H., Van Staalduinen, S., Lemer, C., Greaves, F., Noble, D., Ellis, B., Donaldson, L., & Barraclough, B. (2010). The WHO patient safety curriculum guide for medical schools. *Quality and Safety in Health Care, 19*(6), 542–546. https://doi.org/10.1136/qshc.2009.036970.

World Health Organization. (2010). *International Classification for Patient Safety for Use in Field Testing in 2007–2008 (ICPS)*. WHO.

Index

F

G

H

I

J

K

L

M

N

O

P

Q

R

S

T

U

V

W

www.ingramcontent.com/pod-product-compliance
Lightning Source LLC
LaVergne TN
LVHW071223011026
849280LV00007B/41
* 9 7 8 9 8 1 9 8 2 6 1 5 5 *